Any Woman Can!

Visit Sheila Grant's website at
www.anywomancan.net

Any Woman Can!

How to Get a New Look and a New Life

by SHEILA GRANT
with ANDREA THOMPSON

PARAVIEW PRESS

NEW YORK

Book and cover design by Smythtype
Cover Photo by Klaus Lucka

ISBN: 1-931044-33-3

Library of Congress Catalog Card Number: 2001097767

ANY WOMAN CAN is dedicated to every woman who has dreamed of changing her life, but short of courage, has believed change is impossible.

Beyond myself
somewhere
I wait for my arrival.
            —Octavio Paz

Be it true or false, how we are perceived often has as much influence on our lives, and especially upon our destinies, as what we do.
            —Victor Hugo

Table of Contents

Introduction

I think I know who you are. I don't know your name, of course, or where you live or exactly what you look like, but I am guessing:

You're in your forties, fifties or sixties.

You are, perhaps, romantically unattached—never married (not through any wish of your own), divorced, or moving out of a relationship that has failed. Maybe you've been climbing a career ladder for years, putting everything else on the backburner, and you woke up one day to wonder if it was too late for romance, love and marriage.

You are, perhaps, in a marriage or a relationship that's wrong, maybe even terribly wrong. But the idea of leaving, of being on your own and alone, is terrifying. You may think you don't have the courage or the strength to change and find something better, or you may think it's just too late.

Possibly, you're comfortably married and have been so for years, but those years have been filled with work, raising kids, maintaining a home, keeping the gears of a complicated life oiled and running. *You*—how you looked, how you felt about yourself, what you needed—came last on the list. And the years are showing now, in your body, your face. Your man is still looking youthful. You're looking old.

You're not happy with your appearance. Or, you absolutely hate the way you look. You really know you ought to get to work on yourself, you even know how you should do that—but you're not doing it.

You're not happy with your life. But you think all your chances for a better one have come and gone. It's just too late for you to change.

Am I right?

Now, the good news: You've got a hold of this book. The tide is about to turn!

Let me tell you a little about how this book came to be:

In 1990, I created **Grant Image**, a personal image consulting business—my pride and joy and life's work—and since then I have successfully reimaged over five hundred women (and a fair number of men as well). I lead my client through all the steps she needs to look and feel her best, to dress appealingly, and to present herself with confidence and self-assurance. Time and time again, I have watched my clients begin to take charge of their lives in the most astounding ways. They go after jobs they previously believed were beyond their capabilities; they forge healthier, stronger relationships with the individuals in their lives; they essentially develop their personalities, much for the better.

A couple of years ago, a woman came to me for a consultation. She explained that she'd spent the last twenty years of her life building a business. It was a highly successful business, at that—she had recently sold her company for twenty-three million dollars! She was intelligent, hard-working and determined. Yet she was unhappy and desperately lonely. In her early forties, she hadn't had a date in years. "I always had the attitude," she said, "that this is me, successful and smart. People are going to like me no matter how I look." Maybe people liked her, but men didn't want to take her out and get to know her. She was thinking she should just give up on the idea of ever finding a husband; men, she said, just weren't attracted to her.

I had to be honest with her: Understandably, they wouldn't be! Overweight, frumpy, she looked ten years older than she was. Her hair was bushy and grew low on her forehead, she'd never worn makeup, and her smile revealed lots of gums and yellowish teeth. She dressed like a hippie. Working to achieve independence and success, acquiring more money than she knew what to do with, she hadn't spent any time on herself in years! She had assumed that the right man would somehow, sooner or later, just show up. He hadn't.

By the end of our talk, she'd made a decision to change her life, starting that day. I assured her there was a lovely, attractive woman hiding under all that hair and sadness, dying to be set free. But if we were to be successful, she would have to trust me, and put the same kind of time and effort into her reimaging as she had put into her business. And so the process began.

I helped her reimage herself from the top of her head to her toes. It took months, and relentless determination on her part to lose weight, and to accept and act on all the changes I recommended. Some she resented and protested, such as the suggestions to have her teeth laminated and her gums surgically raised (she did). Together we worked out the plan and I gave her some options. All she had to do was to act on them. None of it was easy.

The remarkable next chapter: A year later, she was, indeed, a beautiful woman. Not only was she lovely to look at; she was, in fact, breathtaking! She moved and talked and interacted with people with a social ease and confidence she had never known. She was meeting men and dating and, she said, "having the time of my life!"

Her story—beginning with my reimaging program—was the subject of a front page article in the Wall Street Journal. Publishers wanted to hear more, and my client went on to write a book about her experiences. And I started to think, again, about something that had been in the back of my mind for years. It was time to write my own book about reimaging. I knew so much I wanted to share with other women, because the journey I've guided hundreds of clients through is a journey I first took myself.

It's a journey that has two parts: First, work hard to get yourself looking and feeling wonderful. Second, work hard to find your life's partner.

When I was first thinking about what I wanted to say, I searched the bookstore shelves to see what else was available for women with the needs I hoped to address. And what I found was most interesting: An armful of books that tell you how to get a man. Yes! In just those words! There's even one of the popular *Idiot's* guidebooks devoted to dating, advising the reader on everything from how to flirt to when to call it quits. Quite a few of these books talk to the older woman; they offer the hopeful message, "love and marriage with the right man can be yours at age forty, fifty and more." They are filled with advice about first dates, communicating, having (or not having) sex, and so on. And somewhere around page 150 is buried the suggestion that a woman searching for romance, love and marriage of course needs to "look good...present a pleasing, attractive appearance."

I found another armful of books about looking great, putting your best image forward, losing weight, dressing in style, and so on and so on. And somewhere around page 150 of *those* books comes the suggestion that all this of course will increase your appeal to men. Or maybe that thought isn't even mentioned at all: Just look great for yourself.

What I'm here to say is, the two go together! The woman who longs to find a terrific man, which is just what so many women I've come to know really do want, in their heart of hearts, must first look and feel like a terrific woman. This is my point of view, and this is how I've put together the book you're about to read. I will show you how to reinvent your appearance, feel great about yourself, and find a healthy, happy relationship with the love of your life. If, however, a new man is not what you need, take your new self and go after your other lifelong dreams and goals.

You can do it. Any woman can.

So let's begin!

PART I
Reimaging Your Way to the Self You Want to Be

In the following two chapters, I want to do two things:

First, I will tell you what changing an image is all about, and why I believe it is so difficult for many women to begin the process.

And second, I'll share with you something about myself—where I started from, what I went through, and what I'm like today. Because I know that if I could change my looks and my life, so can you change yours.

CHAPTER 1

Getting Started, Right Now

Hi Sheila. A friend of mine told me about your reimaging program. I don't know if I need a new image or a new job. Maybe I need a new car! Or a new city! I definitely need a new man! Anyway, I've had a moment of truth recently, and I could use some advice, and I'd like to come in to see you. Help!

That was a message on my machine one day, and soon Amy, the caller, and I were sitting in my living room talking about that "moment of truth." Amy was forty-seven, and divorced for ten years. She was a bank vice president and the mother of a nineteen-year-old son. She said: "This just hit me the other day. You know how men, attractive men, sort of give a woman the eye when they walk past you on the street? Well, I was watching a nice-looking guy walking toward me, and he didn't give me a glance. These days men don't even glance for one second to find out if I'm worth giving the eye. It's like I emit an aura of undesirability! It's like I've become invisible!"

"Do you want men to look at you?" I asked. Amy hesitated. Finally, she said: "I always hoped to remarry. I guess right now I'd just like to meet a sweet guy and spend some enjoyable times together and not feel like I'm out of contention all together."

She dated a bit for a few years after her divorce, but hadn't had a "real romance" in eight years. Being a single mother and working had absorbed all her energies. Her social life revolved around her extended family and some good woman friends.

I forged ahead: "Are you happy with the way you look?" She thought she looked "okay," Amy said. She didn't like "elaborate" clothes; she liked to feel "comfortable." She hated wearing a lot of makeup.

So I forged yet further ahead, and I told this lovely, accomplished, unhappy woman what I tell all the women I work with, and what I'm telling you right now, before we begin: Okay is not good enough! You must look in the mirror on your way out of the house to work in the morning or to a social function at night or just to the neighborhood restaurant for dinner with some pals, and you must smile in delight at what you see there. You must look in the mirror and feel sensational!

Are you looking in the mirror and feeling less than sensational? And why do you have so much company (and trust me, you do!) among women in their forties, fifties and beyond?

I have a theory that goes like this: Somewhere after our thirties, we women lose the ability and the desire to really look at ourselves. We look at other women all the time—at their clothes, their hair cuts, where they fall on the slim-to-chunky-to-fat scale. When it comes to ourselves, we don't look, or we look only in bits and pieces. We look at our mouths in the mirror in order to apply lipstick. We look at our eyes to get the mascara on. Our bodies we generally avoid, except to take a quick glance at the bottom of the mirror on the way out the door, to make sure the hem of the skirt isn't crooked.

Which is one of the reasons why, I think, so many women never figure out how to pull it all together. We don't see ourselves clearly, we don't confront the truth, we tell ourselves we're "okay."

Here's another reason for the Invisible Woman syndrome. When you're twenty-five or thirty, you don't need to do a lot of fussing with your looks. You *can* if you want to. The fussing is fun, it's exciting, but it's not absolutely necessary in order to present yourself to the world as attractive, youthful and desirable. It's not necessary because you've got twenty-five-year-old skin and hair and a twenty-five-year-old body going for you already. When you're forty-five, fifty or fifty-five, on the other hand, you *do* need fussing with your looks. You need more maintenance and artifice, because naturally youthful isn't there anymore. You're neglecting that reality, however, because you're not really looking in the mirror.

We do not do what we have to do to bring out the fabulous, unique, sexy woman inside.

That's what you and I are going to accomplish, starting today, starting now.

Maybe, like Amy and so many of the other women I have advised in my consulting business over the years, you are eager to re-fashion yourself into someone a man sees as appealing, intriguing, inviting; a woman he wants to get to know better. That means a woman he likes the sight of during *the first fifteen seconds* he's met her. (Actually, some studies say that first impressions are cemented within the first seven seconds.)

Fixate briefly on that notion: the fifteen-second window. We will be returning to that thought again and again in this book. It's a powerful notion, and a rather unsettling, irritating, even infuriating one. A man you have never met before will decide on the spot if he likes what he sees and hears, or doesn't much like what he sees and hears. Fifteen seconds is all you have to proceed past stage one, to the point at which he can start to get to know you and you can start to get to know him. If you don't pass muster right then, right there, you must assume there will be no second chance. Call it unfair, call it deplorable, call it superficial, but that's the God's honest truth. So to start, image is everything.

Maybe you are a married woman who senses your marriage is

turning a little stale, because you've "let yourself go." Such was the case with Marianne, a forty-four-year-old mother of two toddlers, who devoted her life to her babies in their comfortable suburban community. When she first came to me for help, Marianne told me she hadn't bought new clothes in five years, hadn't lost her post-pregnancy weight, she cut her own hair to save time, and felt her lawyer husband was losing interest in her. I spent some time with Marianne in her home. We went through her closets and tossed out almost everything. We took a trip to the outlet shops and bought a new wardrobe on sale. I taught her how to accessorize, how to apply makeup, how to style her hair. The upshot: Marianne walked into her husband's office to pick him up for dinner one early evening, and for the first time his partners looked up, smiled, and greeted her enthusiastically. Marianne was no longer the Invisible Woman. After that dinner, her husband suggested they stay out a little longer and go dancing.

Perhaps, like many of my clients, you sense that presenting a more defined, elegant, up-to-date appearance will add to your confidence in your work life or other activities. For example, there was Alice, a manager at a home furnishings warehouse, part of a national chain. At our first meeting, Alice said she suspected she was repeatedly passed over for promotion to regional supervisor, a position that would require traveling and some public speaking, because she didn't look the part. She thought she needed "a more sophisticated appearance," but didn't know how to get one. Together, we added fresher-looking, more stylish separates and accessories to her basically good wardrobe of suits and well-tailored dresses. Alice lightened her hair and got a new cut, and spent a little time practicing what I call "the presentation"—improving her posture and walk, modulating her voice. And yes, Alice got her promotion.

Or perhaps you have stayed with the same "look" for years,

and you're bored. Or maybe you have been noting your changing appearance—arms getting a little flabbier, hair getting a little skimpier—and you keep telling yourself, "All right, I'm aging, this is what happens, just accept it, girl." But secretly, you hate that.

Don't accept it! Without even knowing what you look like at this moment, I guarantee that you can look infinitely better. But getting there is not necessarily going to be fun—not at first, any-way—and definitely will not be easy. You are going to have to become totally committed to the process, even a bit obsessed by it. You must make it your cause, a work to be accomplished, a new job that you are going to take very, very seriously. You must spend time (as much as you have) and money (as much as you can) on this new job. You must pay careful attention to the small-est detail of how you present yourself to the world.

Right about now, you are probably thinking to yourself, "Oh, please! Give me a break!"

How do I know that? Most of the women I've worked with as a consultant put up a great deal of resistance to this idea of obses-sive devotion to the reimaging cause. We over-forty women think it's a little unseemly or adolescent to focus so single-mindedly on appearance. We've been there, done that, and we've left far behind us now the years of self-absorption. Maybe we think there's not much point any more. And maybe, faced with those inevitable changes to our bodies, we comfort ourselves with some old saws—appearances don't count, beauty is skin deep, feel good about yourself on the inside and you'll look good on the outside, and so on and so on. A fantastically gorgeous forty-plus model writes in her beauty book: "I believe that beauty comes from within... My success has been more about who I am than what I look like." Sounds good, but I don't believe it for a minute—and I'll bet she really doesn't either.

We have a slightly schizophrenic attitude about looking great, we over-40s. We want it, but we think it shouldn't count, or not for much anyway. Our other sterling qualities, such as our accomplishments, our smarts, our compassionate natures, our wisdom from our years in the world, should be what make people love us.

Listen to my friend Amy again, as she and I talked over this matter of looks versus sterling qualities. She quoted a line from a Robert Parker detective novel she'd just finished: "Spenser, every woman's ideal guy because he's smart and sensitive and so incredibly macho at the same time, is having drinks with a female friend of his, a lawyer, and he thinks to himself, 'She wasn't beautiful, but her face had in it such intelligence and decency that it may as well have been beautiful.'" Amy went on, with a little self-conscious laugh: "I'm intelligent and decent, so I may as well be beautiful?"

After pointing out to Amy that although Spenser may admire the lawyer, he's powerfully in love with his girlfriend Susan, who's intelligent, decent and absolutely luscious-looking, I acknowledged Amy's sterling qualities and then asked her to consider how they were housed: Shoulder-length, no-name-brown hair with bangs, the way she's "always worn it," she said. A pale face with something too shiny on her lips. A no-nonsense gray suit over a white shirt, what Amy described as "business-casual," (a.k.a., conservative-to-boring.) No-nonsense rubber-soled shoes, comfy footware good for running around in.

Amy does indeed look "okay," but a head-turner she is not. And, as I hope you have now embraced as your mantra: "Okay" is not good enough.

"Okay" is not good enough if you want to continue to charm the delightful man you already have, if you want to infuse your marriage or relationship with new-found satisfaction and fire, because you feel better about yourself as a woman.

"Okay" is not good enough if you want to wake up each

morning anticipating with pleasure the prospect of getting dressed and doing your hair and your makeup, and sailing forth into your day and whatever it may bring.

Most of all, "okay" is definitely not good enough if you want to entice a good man into your life. Not just any man, but a truly fine, decent man who'll take the time and effort to discover all those sterling qualities you possess. If you are unattached, I'm guessing (whether you're ready to say it out loud or not) that *is* what you want, because almost every last one of the hundreds of never married or divorced women I've talked to in my work and in preparing this book have told me they wished for a relationship— someone to share a life with, to grow old with.

I know this woman well.

She is the woman who had no time and space for husband and family during the years of climbing the corporate ladder.

She is the woman who discovered her life partner suddenly had another partner in mind.

She is the woman, like myself, who allowed a man, over many years, to convince her she was not of much worth, who gave up all hope of ever leaving a desperately demeaning, abusive, unhappy marriage because her self esteem was at rock bottom and because she believed all options were closed to her.

She is the woman who thinks she has no way of competing with the twenty-somethings out there. She is the woman who hasn't taken the time to care for herself, who is just plain afraid of change, who resigns herself to a lonely life—or maybe just a mediocre one—out of fear of trying, fear of rejection, fear of failing.

She is the woman who thinks it's too late.

Do you find yourself somewhere in these descriptions? Is some of this ringing a bell with you? If so, this book will change your mind, and if there is one thing I have learned from my own experiences and from my conversations and work with so many women in all walks of life it is this: Reimaging starts with changing how you look. And then, reimaging means changing how you think as well. It means discarding negative thoughts and feelings, deciding that you will not give up, realizing that you can compete and you can be successful and you can find the happiness you want. Reimaging means fixing the outside, and then taking that fabulous self into the world with confidence and starting a whole new life, if that is what you long for.

Looking attractive, feeling good and proud of your image, embracing the power you do possess, will open doors that you may have believed were closed to you forever.

All that can be yours if you decide to commit yourself to the cause. I can make that assurance because the reimaging program I'm going to lead you through is based not only on the experiences of a cross section of women who have followed it, but on my own story and my own success. I know you can do everything I am going to describe because it's a program that works. I know it works because I did it myself—and in the following chapter, I want to tell you a bit about my story, where I started from, what I experienced, and where I am today.

For now, I will just say that my metamorphosis all started with image, as it will for you. I would be the first to admit that change is hard. Almost every woman I have worked with over the past twelve or so years has admitted that acknowledging her dissatisfaction with her looks and life, and then coming to me for help, was one of the most difficult steps she ever took.

Will you enjoy your reimaging program? Will you embrace it willingly? At first, probably not. Inertia is our enemy, the inertia that is the very human response to tackling something different and difficult. We want to put it off. We say we'll get started tomorrow or next year or after the kids leave for college. Often, we try to talk ourselves out of the whole thing. Following some of the recommendations I'm going to make will be a time-consuming effort. You may become impatient, annoyed, resentful that life is not accepting you as you are, that you are reduced to reading a book by a woman you don't even know to get some answers you suspect you need.

But here is a bigger, more insidious mental stumbling block: If you are like many of my clients, you may feel all this we're about to go through is beneath you. It's not fair, not when men can walk around short, bald, slouchy, wrinkled and with hair hanging out of their ears, and *still* be accepted as desirable and powerful competitors, professionally and socially.

I agree with you. You're right, it's downright unfair. Rue it, rail against it, deplore it, write a book about it. Then put all such thoughts out of your mind and go to work.

Something great is about to happen! Small payoffs start coming at once. Bigger payoffs take longer, but are waiting for you in the future. As you begin to look better, your confidence and contentment will grow. And you'll see, you are going to love what you're doing.

Are you ready? I hope so. I'm genuinely excited that you have decided to give me a chance to lead you through your personal reimaging program. And I promise, I will not disappoint you. More importantly, *you* will not disappoint you.

If you looked at my photograph on the jacket of this book, perhaps you thought to yourself something along these lines: "Well, Sheila Grant is a nice-looking woman. Maybe she's had some plastic surgery (I have). Probably that's a professional photograph (it is). Even so, she obviously came into the world looking pretty good to start with. Nobody ever thought she was a plain Jane. And she looks like a confident person too, someone who's made it, who's got what she wants. So how can she have any real appreciation or real sympathy for what my life is like, what I'm going through?"

Before we start the program, I hope you will read the following chapter. In it, I will tell you about my personal journey. It's a journey that began over twenty years ago, when I was in a desperately unhappy place, emotionally and psychologically battered, feeling powerless and trapped and ugly. To write about that time has been painful. But when you have heard my story, you will know something about the passion and experience I bring to my work.

In my years as an image consultant I have guided hundreds of women through some remarkable transformations. What I believe makes me uniquely qualified to write this book, however, and to guide you through your own transformation, has much more to do with my personal story than with what I do professionally. I know exactly what it takes in determination, effort, time and courage to reinvent a life that is unsatisfying, or less than fully lived, or even painful. I know, because that's a road I traveled myself.

And you will understand why I say that if I could change my life, you can change yours. If I could do it, any woman can.

CHAPTER 2

My Story...and Why I Want You to Hear It

One day years ago, I stood in front of a full-length mirror in my bedroom, took a long, hard look at my face, and hated what I saw. The woman in the mirror looked depressed, frumpy, dried up. I lowered my robe and took a long, hard look at my naked body. Neglected, uncared for, unused, unloved.

I was forty-two years old. Many people would have said I was attractive—I was tall, relatively slim, with shapely legs, high cheekbones. The point is, I didn't see a good-looking woman, not even a remotely pretty one. Instead, I saw an insecure, pitiful woman who had lived for years with a husband she feared—a handsome and professionally successful man who convinced her she was worthless; a man who addressed her as "Stupid," not as "Sheila." At that point in my life, I was literally almost unable to function. I could not speak a single sentence without stuttering. I woke up each morning with a feeling of dread for the day to come. I hadn't had sex in years, and hardly considered myself a woman any longer.

The day before that morning when I stared at myself in the mirror, I had just learned that my husband had for years been living a double life, keeping other women, betraying me even as he attempted to destroy me. I had married young, and for most of that time, even after it was clear that little by little I was losing myself, I wanted and clung to the life I had. I never saw myself as anything other than mother, wife, homemaker. It was my entire identity.

On that morning, when making a cup of coffee for myself took all the energy and attention I could summon, I was clearly in the early stage of a nervous breakdown. I looked at the woman in the mirror, and wondered who she was. Where had she been all this time? Who was this woman who for more than twenty years had let a psychologically abusive man suck out of her all feelings of self-esteem, confidence and worth?

Then, at the end of that long, painful session before my mirror, I started to smile. I still cannot really explain why. I don't know whether it was an epiphany or God or just me, finally waking up after years and years, but I smiled. Sensing that I had reached the absolute bottom of the barrel of my life, suddenly it seemed there was nowhere to look but up and out. Staring at my face in the mirror, I said out loud, "Sheila Grant, don't you get it? You don't have to look like this! You don't have to feel like this! You don't have to live like this! You can change!" That was the day I ended my marriage, the day I finally started to emerge from a long nightmare, and the day my metamorphosis began.

But that metamorphosis was a slow, agonizing process, filled with twists and turns. It did not come easily, and it took years. At the start, I had nothing but my children. I was virtually penniless, a woman with no office or business skills. No one, I thought, would find a reason to hire me. And certainly no man would find me attractive, or ever want me. There were still appallingly bad, even frightening times ahead. There were missteps and steps backward. Some of the choices I made, especially regarding men, were unfortunate, to put it mildly.

This is the story of that journey. The particulars of it are unique to me, and yet I believe my situation was far from uncommon. And as you'll see, it has a marvelously happy ending!

TROUBLESOME BEGINNINGS

Matthew Grant was wonderful. He told me so the first time he called. "But I'm handsome, rich, athletic, intelligent, nice, sensitive, funny and an expert handball player. How can you resist?" said this deep, strong masculine voice over the phone, after I had begged off from the blind date a mutual friend was trying to arrange. I had never encountered such arrogance, but at the same time his persistence and apparent confidence was piquing my interest. And the voice was appealing. "Believe me, I'm different from any man you'll meet," he added, and so I agreed to dinner.

I was twenty, and had recently arrived in—or escaped to— New York from a dismal home life in North Carolina. I was working as a showroom model for a dress designer during the day and taking college classes in the evenings. My usual company was the TV, which I switched on as soon as I came into my small midtown apartment. A little lonely but determined to make something of myself, I had no time for men, especially blind dates. But this self-described handsome, funny, sensitive, etc. man intrigued me.

Handsome he was. Tall, well-built, with a strong angular face and pale green eyes, short cropped hair, Matthew looked vaguely like a combination of Warren Beatty and Charlton Heston, but a badly-dressed one, in a ratty jacket and scuffed shoes. The rest of the description didn't hold up on that first date. We went to a dumpy restaurant, ate a mediocre meal in virtual silence. Making conversation with this stranger sitting across from me was extremely difficult—except when he talked about himself, which he obviously liked to do.

He had started his own small company right out of college, vowed to make his first million by age twenty-five, reached that milestone on schedule (he was twenty-six), and was proud of his accomplishments. I liked this fact, that he had determined to be successful, and at such a young age. (Just like my father, a man of the same mold. A man who needed success and money. A man, however, who killed himself when he no longer had success and money, leaving his family destitute.) Matthew Grant was pleased with himself, and apparently pleased with me too. When I declined date number two for the following day, he warned me he was "not a man who gives up easily." For myself, all I knew was that I was very happy to get home to my little apartment, get into bed, hold onto Humphy, my childhood teddy bear, fall asleep, and forget my puzzling evening out.

Early the next morning I received a telegram: I'M CRAZY NUTS ABOUT YOU! LOVE, MATTHEW. And so started a ferocious courtship: phone calls, flowers, telegrams, stuffed animals. A month after this barrage began, I said okay to lunch, and this time was magic time. Now Matthew appeared looking splendid, in a beautiful navy, pin-stripe suit, shined shoes, with a Florida tan and a wide smile. I was totally taken aback by his presence, and I knew at that moment I was in serious trouble. We went to an elegant restaurant, drank champagne, and talked non-stop for hours, about anything and everything. Later, we walked hand and hand through a snowy Central Park, and stopped and kissed and held each other. I was smitten—totally, thoroughly, positively in love. Just like that.

Clearly Matthew Grant knew how to get what he wanted. And now he wanted me. And he had me. I moved in with him the following week, and I had never been so happy in my life. We traveled, we laughed, we loved, and except for that last part, the loving, everything was perfect.

Sex was unsatisfying. Although I felt sure of this man's feelings for me, he never said "I love you" when we were in bed together, never made me feel sensual and special and safe. Instead, he became cold, detached, as if he were making love to a stranger. It became clear that I was there for the purpose of pleasing him.

Later, though, he'd hold me, kiss me, stroke my hair.

How did I feel about all this? Disappointed, certainly. Confused. I tried to talk about our sexual relationship, but such talk upset him. This was a man, I was discovering, who could become moody, angry and withdrawn if he was questioned, if things were not going the way he wanted them to. I had never enjoyed a good sexual relationship before, and really had no basis of comparison. I thought that maybe what my mother always told me was right, that sex is what you have to put up with to please a man. Don't expect to like it, don't expect to be happy, don't expect to feel loved. So I made excuses to myself for his difficult behavior. I told myself that all would change over time, of course it would. I knew I didn't want to be alone. I was just going to make this work. It was up to me.

After we'd been living together for some months, I broached the "M" word and Matthew immediately said he never wanted to get married. In fact, he became almost violent on the subject. He told me he did want to live with me, probably forever, but not as husband and wife. I wouldn't want "to ruin a perfectly good relationship," would I? More denial on my part: Of course he didn't mean it, all men are nervous about marriage, I just had to be patient. There followed months of my "being patient," until one day I gave up, packed my belongings and moved back in with my old roommate. It would be the most difficult time of my life thus far. I ached as I had never ached for anyone. I cried, I mourned the death of a relationship I had worked so hard to keep and the loss of the man I loved with all my being.

Then one day, I got a phone call. It was Matthew, insisting he couldn't live without me, telling me he did want to marry me, he had his mother's ring waiting for me. And I went from crying in despair to crying for joy, from filling my hours with work to planning my wedding. It would be small and elegant—and soon! I insisted we marry immediately, no doubt having an inkling that he might change his mind. But Matt seemed genuinely happy for the first time in our relationship. He was kinder, more loving. All would, at last, be well. So I fervently believed.

All was far from well, and if God was sending me a message to run the other way, the signs were powerful indeed. The day before my wedding—in fact, just as I was trying on the beautiful white, satin and lace gown the designer I worked for had made for me—I noticed that the joints in my right arm and left leg were red and swollen. I felt exhausted and feverish. When Matthew arrived home from work, I told him I wasn't feeling well, and not up to dinner out as we had planned. He replied that was fine with him, because he wasn't feeling all that great himself. Looking anxious and jumpy, he seemed to be having a touch of a nervous breakdown! Impending nuptials apparently weren't agreeing with his nervous system. This marriage was off to some start.

As it turned out, my temperature climbed to an alarming degree, and I was rushed to the emergency room. At first I was diagnosed with rheumatic fever, and told I'd be in bed for a year. Then I was advised I had "a rare unknown virus," and spent ten days in the hospital before my fever, swelling and stiffness subsided. One week later, I talked Matthew (actually, make that threatened him) into marrying me, fast. And there we were, standing before a justice of the peace, me not in my satin gown but in a pink suit, pink stockings, pink shoes, with deep, dark circles under my eyes and a jaundiced yellow glow to my face (I clashed with everything) and Matthew in the ratty sports jacket he had worn on our first, unpleasant date, looking sick, depleted and angry.

It was a perfectly awful day from beginning to end. At our "wedding dinner" in the dining room of the "Motel on the Mountain," my brand new husband did more drinking than dining, and had to be helped by the manager back to our honeymoon suite. I remember still the look on that man's face as he dropped Matt's leaden body onto the bed: "You got yourself a real doozy, didn't you young lady?"

What had I done to my life?

NEWLYWEDS FROM HELL

"Mrs. Matthew Grant." I had the wedding license to prove it. Sometimes I took out that license and stared at it, for confirmation, because in most other respects, I didn't feel anything like a married woman, a wife, a lover of the man I loved. We had no sex. Exchanged no signs of affection. We lived in Matt's apartment, a place he had clearly designed to be a "bachelor pad," complete with pushbutton-controlled lights, fancy stereo, and a very large jacuzzi. Evidences of other women—two lipsticks, not my shade, some hair clips, not mine, stuck behind the aspirin bottles in the cabinet—were still about. Women called occasionally. Neither he nor I ever mentioned the dismal wedding; it was as if none of it had ever happened.

What had I expected? Matt had told me—warned me, in fact—that he did not want to be married. What had I been thinking? *Had* I been thinking?

As the weeks passed, enormously painful and difficult weeks, I reverted to my old pattern. I did everything I could possibly think of to please this husband of mine, to turn things around and make him happy. And nothing seemed to matter! He was distant, obviously depressed, often belligerent. Sometimes his face was twisted with guilt and pain. Clearly, he didn't know what to do with me. He *had* loved me, of that I was sure. Still, Matthew never attempted to make love to me, kiss me or hold me. I begged him to talk to me about our situation, explain to me what was happening so I could help. His reply was simply: "I told you I couldn't be married. I'm working on it. I need time."

I was trying to deal with my enormous insecurities and self-doubts, now hitting all time highs. And still, I kept thinking: It must be me! I must have done something wrong, but what? I really didn't know, and that was slowly but surely destroying me and whatever self esteem I had left. It took everything in me not to fold up and run for my life. Or is this "just men?" Was Matthew cheating on me? Do all men? My father cheated on my mother the day after they were married, she once told me. I remembered the sight of my mother washing lipstick stains off Daddy's shirt collars, tears spilling from her eyes into the sink.

One evening two friends surprised us with a "wedding party." Arriving at their home for a quiet dinner for four, thirty-five friends and acquaintances burst from the other room to greet Matthew and me, champagne glasses in hand, toasting us. It was a beautiful party, with wonderful food, flowing champagne, great music, everyone congratulating us and saying what a handsome couple we made. And me, the happy bride? I was in shock.

I discovered something that evening: I was quite good at play-acting. Maybe another career awaited me after this nightmare! I smiled, I talked, I played the part of the blissful newlywed, and it was a perfectly awful time for me.

The day I decided to put an end to this strange life I had entered was the day I showed up unannounced at Matt's office and found him with a woman—a rather large-breasted redhead. She was naked. So was he. Both jumped off the couch like scared rabbits as I stared, speechless. Then I quietly closed the door and left. By the end of that day I had moved in with my friend Patty. By the following day, thanks to Patty, I had found a wonderful lawyer and then an equally wonderful psychologist.

It would be weeks before I could eat without feeling as if I would throw up. Weeks during which I would wake up in the middle of the night in a cold sweat, seeing my husband make love to another woman, the husband who wouldn't make love to me. An enormous amount of damage had occurred. I felt a genuine revulsion towards men. But with my therapist's help, I began the arduous task of delving into my past to unveil the patterns my life seemed to be taking. I saw that in my desire to be needed and loved, I had made compromises in ways I could never have imagined. And I saw too that the man I had married suffered from a kind of sickness, one not all that uncommon, in which a wife becomes somehow confused with an untouchable mother figure—whore/slut before marriage, madonna/mother after marriage. I began to think, yes, I'm going to survive this.

And that should have been the beginning of the beginning. But it wasn't.

Matthew refused to sign the annulment papers my lawyer had sent him (I had asked for only enough money to pay my therapist and get back on my feet). The courtship began again—the flowers, phone calls, letters. Experiencing a new if still shaky sense of strength and control, I ignored it all. Six months to the day I left, Matt appeared kneeling at my door, flowers in hand, looking drawn and teary, like a little boy who had done something quite terrible and wanted forgiveness. He loved me so much, he said, he really hoped we would be able to have a normal marriage. He knew he had problems, but he wanted a home, a wife, me. We'd get married again, "the right way this time." We'd go to a psychiatrist together, and he'd found one he believed could help him. We'd sell the apartment and live anywhere I wanted. If only I'd give him one more chance.

I gave him that chance. We'd live together for one month, I told him, on a trial basis. If, by some remote possibility, it worked out, I would stay. If it did not, he was to give me an immediate divorce and we'd part for good. Crying, holding me, Matthew thanked me over and over, saying he'd make me "the happiest woman in the world."

Did I believe it would work? Not really. Still, one more chance to have what I had wanted more than anything in life seemed like the right gamble to take.

Looking back on that day and that decision has brought me many regrets. I had a moment of strength back then that I wouldn't experience again for a long, long time. I had the opportunity, right then, to save the next twenty years of my life. But I was only twenty-two years old. I believed there was hope for my husband, that by admitting his problem he could change. I still loved him. And women can be fools for the men they still love.

Surprisingly, Matthew began fulfilling his promises immediately. We saw a psychiatrist the first day we were back together. There I began to hear the full, shocking measure of the demons this man faced. His childhood in many ways was as appallingly painful and confusing as mine had been. I tried to understand, tried to accept, wanted to believe there was hope. And so we began the process of working on the problems that had destroyed our first attempt at marriage. I threw myself into the role of becoming the perfect wife. I took cooking lessons, made my husband's favorite dishes, created a comfortable home in our new apartment. It made me happy to make him happy. That was my job. Sometimes I thought about a "real" job, but Matthew declared, "I don't want my wife to work. I want you home."

In time, the sessions with the psychiatrist dropped off. My ability to please my husband seemed not to be working so well. I found myself attacked at every chance he got. At dinner parties or other settings in front of people, he seemed to enjoy making me feel foolish, ignorant, and inept. (Just like my father, a man I could never please, a man who called me "ridiculous," "silly," "ugly.")

There were "boys' nights out" and "dinners with clients." Asking about any of this only resulted in more attacks, more confrontations, more shouting. Suddenly, when I tried to speak I stuttered, something I'd never done before. Slowly, surely, I was reaching new levels of insecurity that left me with this embarrassing affliction, which made my husband laugh. We had no sex. We never kissed. I asked myself how I felt about this man I married, and I discovered I still loved him, needed him, depended on him— but I didn't like him. Actually, I had started to fear him.

There were some rewards. Matthew was becoming enormously successful. Money, as the saying goes, was no object. I had struggled for so many years, working since I was thirteen to help support my mother and sister. Now I could have almost anything I wanted. When I felt especially miserable and despondent, I could go shopping! Sometimes, it actually worked. After a little spree, I'd forget my problems for a bit and feel an enormous high, but that was always followed by an equally enormous low. The price I paid for the good life was a great one.

Sometimes I pulled away. I felt a bit more courageous and able to think a bit more clearly, and realized I simply couldn't and wouldn't live like this anymore. My husband always sensed those times when the end was about to come, and abruptly would tell me: "I do love you. I never want to be without you. Hang in there. I know it hasn't been easy. I'll try harder. Give me one more chance."

So it went. Always one more chance, always trying to believe a miracle would occur. I cooked, I shopped, I took up sculpting, I made friends. And one day I woke up and I was twenty-nine years old. I felt like a foolish woman, empty, useless, unloved. I wanted a child.

How does a married woman go without any sex whatsoever for seven years? I had done it by blocking it out, turning off the switch, obliterating all thoughts and fantasies of love-making. My husband did love me, he insisted, and he wanted to give me a baby, he said now. But I would have to make some accommodations to his needs.

I will only say that I devised my own ways of being the whore of his fantasies. To get what I wanted, I played a game that appalled me. It was a game that caused me the most profound humiliation and guilt. "God knows every sin we commit," I heard my mother's voice telling me. "Remember, He knows everything...don't ever disappoint him...don't do anything you wouldn't want God to see!" We didn't make love; we had sex. Part of me believed it was all worth it—destroying my self-respect, feeling debased; part of me believed having a child would change everything, would enable us to have a normal marriage.

Our daughter was born—our perfect, splendid, beautiful daughter. We needed a house, my husband said now, a real home, and so he simply went out (not consulting me) and bought one. So my next job was to become the perfect suburban housewife. But at least I had my child. I know all parents feel they have the most perfect baby in the world, but they're mistaken—I did. She was my joy. But of course, she grew up, and entered school, and so with time on my hands I threw myself into becoming the consummate homemaker. There were more cooking lessons. I gardened, I gave dinner parties, joined a club, the works. But all the while I was becoming more and more withdrawn and depressed. I couldn't speak clearly. When I heard the door open, signaling the arrival of my husband, I curled up, shrunk into myself. Something was happening that was out of my control

Once again, Matthew, who generally never spoke to me except with an insult, accusation or rebuke, pulled me back in. Once again, discussions were underway, negotiating my life: He'd change, we'd take a vacation, we'd have another child. So I played the game once more, and that year—five years after my daughter was born—we had our son, the second most beautiful baby I had ever seen. I immediately fell madly in love and had renewed purpose in life. I was needed.

The children made Matthew happier than I had ever know him to be. I don't believe this driven, desperate man had ever really experienced peace and happiness. His son and daughter came as close to giving him those gifts as anything ever had. I, on the other hand, could do nothing right—except cook. My sculpting became terribly important to my well-being. Chipping away furiously on 300-400 pound stones proved to be an ideal way to relieve pent-up anxiety and despair. My teacher said I had "real talent," and my first piece found its way into a show and took third place. I was proud of my new-found hobby and talent, but my husband wasn't. "What the hell is that?" was his only comment on one of my sculptures.

I was getting older fast. Turning forty, I could hardly avoid thinking about where I was in my life, and where I wasn't. My kids were in school and I was alone again, living in a marriage without intimacy, companionship, sex or love. Would I leave when my children were grown? Would I be too old by then, and maybe not care anymore? Could I ever, in fact, leave? Matthew was traveling a great deal on business in those days, and I cherished the times without him. Was this how it would always be?

I never revealed my great unhappiness to anyone, and even our closest friends had no idea that our marriage was a fraud. Who would have suspected? We had it all. Everyone said so. Such a handsome family!

All the while I was also sinking ever more deeply into depression, finding it harder and harder to get out of bed each day, still unable to speak without stuttering. Oddly, I felt as I had all those years ago on the day before my planned wedding— terribly sick, almost paralyzed. All this made little sense to me. I knew I had many blessings in life. My children were wonderful, I lived in a beautiful house. Still, something was very wrong with me.

Over the years, off and on, Matthew and I had seen a psychologist in an effort to "work on our problems." These sessions, however, petered out quickly and resulted in nothing. One day, completely uncharacteristically, I broke down during lunch with a close friend, and admitted to her some of my despair. This dear woman gave me the best advice I could have heard at that point— I needed professional help, and from someone who didn't know Matthew. I took that advice, saw "my own" psychiatrist for the first time since early in my marriage, and gave this helpful individual a broad look at what the past two decades had been like. At the end of that session, I heard from him something I hadn't wanted to hear: I was the one with the problems, he suggested. I had allowed everything that happened to happen. No one had made me stay. Only I could change my life.

Not long after that meeting, I received from a friend who knew my family well, the news that would finally begin my real metamorphosis. It was the news that prompted that long, despairing look at the unhappy woman in the mirror. The news was devastating: There had been other women in my husband's life (over 300 of them, as it turned out), there had been apartments maintained in several cities, there had been attempted seductions of other women in my own home, there had been fake "modeling agencies" that lured in women, and more.

Events happened quickly after that. Appearances, it turned out, were truly deceiving. That wonderful life, the impression that "we had it all," was a sham and was about to come crashing down. My husband's business had failed, important bills hadn't been paid in months. We were, I learned from the lawyers, not only deeply in debt, but actually on the verge of bankruptcy. Money had always been there when nothing else was. Now that, too, was gone. And, having unthinkingly co-signed certain documents my husband had put in front of me, I was personally liable for some of our obligations.

To say I was terrified of the future is an understatement. What about the children? How would we live? Where would we live? How would they deal with the loss of their home, the seeming loss of the father they loved? At the same time, I was angry, angrier than I had ever been in my life. In that final session with the therapist, when I learned all the appalling facts, when there was yet one more pathetic plea for yet "one more chance," I heard this from my husband and I knew it was the truth: I had made it easy for him. He was able to do what he did because I never really wanted to know. Out of some combination of fear, neediness, desperation and hope, I never confronted or questioned, never demanded what was my due not only as a married woman, but as a human being—that is, respect, admiration, intimacy and love.

The anger served me well. I knew I had terribly serious issues to deal with and mammoth problems to solve, but I also knew I was going to be okay. Better than okay. I would have my life back.

Lessons learned

I have described those years, from my so-called courtship through my so-called marriage, in some detail, because I believe they tell a story about change that applies to the lives of many women. The lessons I learned have something to say to *any* woman who sets out on the reimaging path, *any* woman who determines to start now to improve her life. Here's what I think those lessons are:

1) Never allow yourself to accept abusive treatment.

This is my personal crusade, so permit me to get on my soapbox briefly. In all likelihood, you didn't buy this book because you feel trapped in an abusive, destructive relationship. At least, I pray that you did not. You most likely bought this book because you've simply decided you can and want to feel better about yourself—more attractive, more desirable, more polished or confident, which is all to the good. But to any woman who may be living in a bad relationship, I'd like to offer these thoughts:

A close friend—I'll call her Anne—married a man she had known for some time, admired greatly, and came to love. Two months after their elegant wedding, Anne and her husband had an argument one evening, the kind of tiff all couples experience sooner or later. At the height of the argument, Anne's husband suddenly hit her in the face with the back of his hand, hard enough to split her lip, and rammed her against the wall, hard enough to damage her shoulder. The following day she moved out of their apartment. Two weeks after that she served him with divorce papers. "He was not the man I thought he was," Anne told me. Perhaps he could change, she said, perhaps he could root out this apparent tendency for physical violence, but she thought he probably couldn't, and in any case she didn't intend to wait around and be part of the process.

My friend suffered from the loss of her dream, she cried at night for a long time, she listened painfully to her husband's pleas for forgiveness—but she took a clear, swift action that she knew was the right one. She sensed that allowing herself to be sucked into this man's problems was no good for her, and that she would find a better, healthier path. (She did, in marriage to a fine man with whom she now shares a law practice.)

For every Anne, there are a thousand women who choose to stay, and wait year after year for him "to change," or who try to summon up the strength to leave. They are women without money of their own and women with excellent jobs. They are women with children and without children. They are beautiful-looking women or ordinary-looking women; they are young or old.

And many of them, I believe, grew up as little girls who never heard anyone tell them they were good and strong and pretty and lovable. The roots go deep, the damage can be traced way back. I have mentioned here the father who called me dumb, ridiculous, foolish. He never gave me a hug, never said "I love you." *Only once* did he offer a kind word, if it can be called that. We were at the beach. I was eleven years old. It was one year before his suicide. He stared at me for a while, and then said, "Maybe you won't turn out to be as ugly as I thought."

In retrospect, of course, it is crystal clear that I moved from one abusive, demeaning, rejecting man, my father, to another, my husband. And for so long, I saw no way out. It's a familiar story, one I've heard, sadly, from many other women. We're programmed from childhood to take less than we deserve, to be quiet and submissive and afraid to speak up in our own defense. Call it head-in-the-sand behavior, call it denial. Call it fear of change or lack of self-esteem. It is all that, perhaps, but often I think it's something more as well—a deep longing for family and connection. It's the belief that if you just keep trying hard enough, and then try a little harder still, or if you make just one more compromise, you can make things right. I know all those feelings, all those many ways of persuading oneself that there is no other option but to stay.

Each of us must make her own decisions, chart her own path. But I hope that any woman reading this book will realize that there are many forms of abuse. Psychological and emotional abuse, taunting and ridiculing another human being, intentionally setting out to make that individual feel worthless, is every bit as devastating and destructive as the slap, the shove and the punch. Being on the receiving end of persistent, determined psychological abuse wounds the soul and corrodes the will.

If the signs are there, read them and heed them.

2) *As you begin to change your life, one step forward may be followed by two steps back.*

Real change for the better takes determination more than anything else, and determination is a tricky quality to maintain. In my own experience, each time I rallied a bit of gumption and felt ready to move on, forces holding me back—some internal, some external—proved to be stronger.

Progress doesn't always happen in a steady, upward-and-onward flow. You may make mistakes, you may feel stalled at times. Keep the end in mind, and don't allow yourself to become discouraged.

3) *Believe that love is possible for you.*

Love is wonderful! Having a good man in your life is wonderful! If part (or all) of your motivation to reimage yourself is coming from the wish or the hope that you will find love with a good man, say it out loud! If you are longing for a relationship, acknowledge that to yourself!

I've said in the previous sections that I believe most women really want to have a man. It is and should be important that a woman admit this, and not convince herself she can live very nicely without one. Certainly some women prefer life on their own. Based on my own experience, however, and from coming to know hundreds of unattached women in my professional work and in conducting interviews for this book, I am convinced that most of us really do want love, relationship and marriage.

Believe that it is a worthy, normal, understandable goal, and that it is possible for you!

Believing is the starting point. Even at my lowest ebb, when my feelings of self-respect and self-admiration were rock bottom, a small voice inside told me my hope and dream of love was healthy and right. Listen to your own small voice—or get one going if it's not there now! When you believe love is possible, you'll find it a lot easier to turn off the negative, despairing voice that says, "It's just too hard to find a man... there are no good men left out there...my chances have passed me by." And then you'll find the courage and determination to get your reimaging underway. Never let it be too late.

We will say more—much more!—about love and men later.

Up from the abyss

Picture me back then in front of my mirror, looking awful, old, neglected and scared. And at the end, saying, "You don't have to live like this!" I *had* to change. My children needed me. I had to support us, I had to start feeling good about myself.

That same day I began my own reimaging. The woman I saw in the mirror, I could acknowledge, also had some positive things going for her. She had a body in fairly good shape and pretty eyes. Impulsively, arming myself with a drugstore hair coloring kit and my manicure scissors, I spent an hour in the bathroom and emerged with a Nordic Blonde, short, angular cut. (The do-it-yourself haircut I will *not* recommend for you!) The change was underway. The cause had begun.

I'd always had a flair for dressing, or just a sense of what looks attractive and why. I had a good eye, you might say. I could also sew, and when I was younger I had made many of my own clothes. But because I was deeply depressed, all those abilities and assets went by the board. For years I'd been living mainly in warmup suits and sneakers, my hair pulled back in a rubber band just to get it out of the way. Now I went out and worked the credit cards one more time. My legs were shapely; I bought two fabulous outfits that showed them off. I bought new makeup for the first time in years, and I figured out how to play up my eyes and cheekbones.

Sometime after that began a pure fairy tale. It was the miracle I'd been praying for, although a very different one than I had hoped for all those years. I became Ford model.

A photographer acquaintance asked me if I had ever modeled, startling me with his question. It had been years since I'd worked for the dress designer, and in any case I had never posed for photographs. "Would you like to?" he asked. "Well, sure, I guess so, but...," I said, and with that he called the Ford modeling agency and make an appointment for me to meet an agent that afternoon. Ford, it seemed, was looking for "Fabulous and Forty" models at the time, and in what would be one of the biggest surprises of my life I was taken on that same day!

Driving into the city some days later to my very first assignment, a photo shoot for *Harper's Bazaar*, tears poured down my cheeks as I thought about painful realities I had to face. I was a woman who hadn't earned money in years, who had never been "allowed" to have a job, who was now financially responsible for two young children. But that first shoot was magical. I was transformed by makeup stylists and hairdressers into a different woman: I looked beautiful! The people around me were telling me I was beautiful! They said that I was a "natural," and they were right. For some reason, the former frightened, insecure, depressed housewife found she could perform in front of a camera. The pictures proved it. I let go of every inhibition, and just adored that camera and the feelings I was having.

I started then, because I had to, saying, "Yes, I can do this!" Over time, my picture appeared in countless magazines, advertising everything from jewelry and designer clothes to hemorrhoid creams! My children would shriek in delight when they opened a copy of *McCalls*, *Vogue* or another magazine and saw their mommy, looking every inch the glamour puss. They were so proud of me. I was proud of me.

I said, "Yes, I can do this" again months later when, thanks to the prompting and pushing of my oldest and dearest friend Mariette Hartley, I was offered a job as fashion director of the CBS "Good Morning America Program." How I landed such a job I still don't know, offering as I did no resume and no experience. But suddenly I was working ten-hour days and giving it my best shot, knowing that thanks to Mariette I'd been handed an incredible opportunity that just could save my life.

I found myself "dressing" the four stars each morning, and working with guest celebrities, preparing their appearance for the camera. It was beyond exciting, and at the same time, beyond scary! In fact, I must admit I was often winging it! And yet, I was productive. My "good eye" served me well. Little by little I was discovering that I had talents and intelligence, that I was a woman who could take on a hell of a lot more than she ever dreamed.

One day I learned that I would be doing my own on-air beauty segments, the network powers-that-be assuming I knew what I was doing. I definitely didn't, but there I was, on national television, the woman who only a short time earlier could not speak without stuttering. In fact, I never stuttered again after leaving my marriage, but neither was I ready for prime time! It was terrifying! Some days I was sure I couldn't handle it. More days, I had never felt better or stronger in my life.

Being a Ford model and a television commentator, in and of itself, was exhilarating and fulfilling, and I continued to learn an enormous amount from the stylists, makeup artists, photographers and cameramen I worked with. Later, I was hired by NBC and spent two years there as a fashion director. Slowly, I was regaining a measure of self-esteem, and honing some useful skills as well.

Even as something resembling a career began to fall into place, social life was something else. I never had as much physical reimaging to accomplish on myself as I now understand many women do. I *did* have to learn to value my looks and let them show, and to care for myself. But there was a bigger problem: much effort had to go into ridding myself of dreadful patterns acquired over years, especially the need to find the difficult, demeaning, controlling men I thought were all I deserved. I had to reemerge in a social world that terrified me for a long time, and keep fighting back the small demons of doubt and insecurity that were always in the wings. In short, I had to reimage my head. It would take me the better part of ten years.

STARTING A NEW LIFE...AND REPEATING OLD PATTERNS

When the house was finally sold, the children and I moved into a small city apartment. I was working, but we went through a long and arduous period of financial struggle. At times, I worried how we would eat. Debts had to be paid off, the divorce arranged, new schools adjusted to, many emotionally draining and physically exhausting issues to confront. The children hated living in the city, hated me for uprooting their lives. Up at 4:30 a.m., I was at the studios before dawn.

In time, life became a bit calmer and more predictable. And I decided to stick my toe in the social waters, very tentatively, very nervously.

A cocktail party was my first venture out on my own in twenty-three years. It did not feel very good to be a forty-three-year-old mother worrying about what to wear, how to look, what to say. To walk into a room filled with people I didn't know, to suspect I came across with all the confidence of an insecure teenager—it was all too much! The nervousness finally wore off, however, and I began to enjoy myself. Before the evening was over I had been introduced to a charming and attractive (and, I had been told by my hostess) very eligible man, who invited me to lunch on the following day.

My first date in twenty-three years! Again, I found myself stewing about what to wear, what to say. Getting dressed in the morning, I suddenly became obsessed by the fact that all the underwear I owned was white cotton Jockey. I would have to do something about that, get some sexy stuff. Then I asked myself why I was worrying about my underwear for a lunch date!

At the restaurant, trying to exude confidence, I was feeling like a nervous wreck. Over our wine and shrimp salad, I found myself answering Mr. Eligible's questions about my separation and pending divorce, talking a bit about the difficulties of starting this brand new life of mine. "You didn't have affairs while you were married?" he asked suddenly, taking me by surprise. I felt enormously insulted. Was this how all men view women and marriage?

"Of course not," I said, "what a thing to say. Either you're married or you aren't. *You* are my first affair. I mean...of course this isn't an affair...it's a luncheon affair, so to speak...." I babbled on, to my immense embarrassment and his great amusement.

Despite that awkward beginning, we did become lovers, and I luxuriated in the first truly satisfying sexual relationship I had ever had. How wonderful it was to realize that I wasn't a shriveled, dried up, old woman after all. And I was, once again in my life, on the receiving end of a whirlwind courtship—flowers, gifts, exclamations of love. Then, one day when the children were staying with their father, Mr. Eligible planned a glamorous "perfect night" for us in his apartment. There was champagne, an elegant dinner. We laughed and talked until one in the morning. It was perfect. But as he was taking a last sip of cognac from his glass, the tone of the evening took a startling turn. Mr. E's speech changed. He slurred his words so much that his tongue seemed twisted. Suddenly, he threw me down and pinned me tightly to the floor, one hand around my neck. "You won't hurt me, will you?" he was shouting, choking me. "You won't see any other men! Tell me that!"

I was gasping for air, first wondering if this was some kind of bizarre joke, then fighting him off. Raising his other hand as if to strike me, abruptly he fell onto his back, hitting his head on the parquet floor. A shiver of terror shot through me. For a moment, I thought he was dead. About to panic, I heard a sawing noise. He was snoring! Throwing on the rest of my clothes, I ran out, and ran home.

I refused to see Mr. Eligible again. But he was the first in a number of encounters that finally convinced me of something I hadn't been wanting to know: I still needed a man in my life, for all the worst reasons—to prove I was loveable, to tell me I was smart, pretty, desirable. My pattern of finding sick men continued. I would have a lot of work ahead of me.

I met another Mr. Eligible, who spent the first half hour of our dinner at a lovely restaurant visually scanning the room, looking at everyone, especially women, except me. This very handsome man suddenly blurted out, "Normally I never go on blind dates." They seldom work out, he continued, and: "You're very attractive, don't take this personally, but I guess I was expecting someone a lot younger. Not that you're old...." He, as I learned in the course of the strained evening that followed that casual cruelty, was fifty-five.

I worried a lot about looking old, started focusing on every line and wrinkle on my face, the little pouches forming around the sides of my mouth. Soon I caught myself pulling the skin back toward my hairline to see if I looked younger. I started to consider having a facelift. In truth, I had conflicting emotions about the whole idea. We do live in a youth-oriented society, no escaping the fact. And I was competing professionally with women half my age. Looking my youngest had practical consequences. Besides, after years of neglecting my appearance, I now was a firm believer that every woman should feel great about herself, and feeling great has a lot to do with looking good.

And yet, it was mostly about men. I was feeling terribly insecure about my age, worrying about what the lighting would be like in the restaurant I'd be going to. Would it be too bright, too wrinkle-revealing? Was this yet one more thing I'd undertake to please a man? I finally decided to go for it and I had the face lift.

I met men who told me they'd "done the kid thing," and they didn't want to go there again. I met men who actively disliked children. There was one who talked to my kids as if he were conducting a board meeting, his voice and manner intimidating, and who shouted at my daughter when she accidentally knocked a dinner roll on the floor.

Twice I came close to marriage. But again, there I was, still trying to persuade myself that the wrong man was the right man. Both men were handsome, successful, powerful, and offered a promising escape from the financial struggles that always plagued me. At the same time, they were controlling, manipulative and demanding.

I went back to therapy, and this time the process was serious, long and arduous. I spent many hours reviewing patterns I had come to know too well, unveiling problems I hadn't really understood before.

What I realized was that I had no true concept of myself. My self-image was bordering on non-existent. When a successful, intelligent man showed interest in me, I was shocked. I'd wonder, what is a man like this doing with me? I had absolutely no idea of who I was, or what I looked like. My life might have taken a very different turn if I had ever liked myself, just a little. Deep down, I didn't really believe I could take care of myself; I felt I needed to be married. The thought of life on my own filled me with sadness and fear.

But despite all the insecurity, the bad moves when it came to men, and the lessons still to be learned, I wasn't waking up feeling depressed as I had done for years. I woke up excited, hopeful. Sure, I was scared to death sometimes at the reality of raising my kids and earning money, but I was excited to be alive. Sometimes, I wasn't quite sure who this new woman was. She could be uninhibited; she could be outrageous! I had spent my life being the nice girl, always doing the right thing. Maybe it was time for a change.

All along I knew that somehow I was going to be okay. I even believed I'd meet a wonderful man one day and have a normal, real relationship, once I understood why I allowed terrible men into my life.

The over-forty singles scene: Desperately seeking Mr. Right

Over time, I began to acquire a more objective view of this whole business of meeting men. I found myself in a social set of sorts, in which women talked to each other about the newly divorced man who had just "come on the market." I decided to investigate some of the venues single men and women have to meet a partner, and discovered that most were humiliating, disappointing and downright awful!

I went to a singles party, which cost forty dollars to circulate among an array of the lonely and desperate, the bitter, the divorced, the divorced-for-the-evening, the confirmed bachelors, the one-night standers. But it was a way to meet people, said my friend, who advised me to take the "don't-come-near-me-or-I'll-kill-you-look" off my face. It was quite an evening, and I learned a great deal about the singles game.

Some of what I heard amazed me. Women joined AA because there were some great guys at the meetings, or became "born again" because of the terrific singles group at the church. Women took the shuttle to Washington or Boston a couple of times a week at the business hour, hoping to sit next to an available man. They read the obituaries, hoping to spot a fresh widower, hung around in the men's department at Bloomingdale's, and worked out at the Vertical Club in full makeup. The "desperately seeking Mr. Right" list went on and on.

I met lovely unattached women, perfectly sane, normal women who wished to meet men. And I met some others of a very different stripe, the women I came to think of as a school of barracudas. These were women who looked for very rich, very successful men who would give them lifestyles, not necessarily love.

I found it all rather fascinating. Some of it would have even been funny, if it wasn't so enormously sad. Did finding a man have to be this difficult? Was it true that "all the good men are taken?" A man, it seemed, simply had to have a heartbeat and show up. A woman, on the other hand, had to kick and claw and scramble in her search for love. This was a seriously competitive and desperate world I'd never dreamed existed.

Hearing about a professional matchmaker, a woman who claimed responsibility for arranging over 7,000 marriages, I decided to go "undercover," present myself as a candidate for her services, and find out more about the lengths women would go to in order to land a man. Marital happiness, I learned immediately, didn't come cheap—for $25,000, Madame Matchmaker would find you a millionaire husband; $15,000 produced a moderately wealthy one, and the fee was $6,000 for...well, "just a guy." If you were strapped for cash, you could charge Mr. Right on your Visa or Mastercard.

I apologized, explaining that I really couldn't afford to buy a husband at that point in time, and saw Madame studying me thoughtfully. "I tell you what," she said, "you come work for me, I can use your help with some of my customers. You make over the *mesquites*, the uglies. Tell them how to dress, fix their hair, make themselves look better." It was an offer I couldn't refuse. The pay was excellent and the hours were short. Officially a consultant now, I worked with dozens of women who came hoping the matchmaker would bring magic into their lives. There was the very overweight woman who had taken out a substantial loan and was ready to pay every cent she had for that magic. There was the sweet and shy ex-nun who had to find the courage to buy a lipstick for herself. Most of them, if not all, were sad, lonely and desperate.

As you may have guessed, these women were being bilked by the matchmaker, who was revealed to be a total fraud. She was finally indicted and her business was shut down.

I started to think more seriously that maybe I really could do something about all this misery. My modeling assignments were becoming more sporadic, my TV jobs had ended. With a loan from a friend, I took the plunge and started my own company, calling it Re-Image Inc. and then Grant Image. I wanted to help women look and feel better about themselves. I wanted to urge them to consider how they might reinvent their lives. In time, the business thrived! I gave seminars, appeared on many TV shows, even was offered my own cable show, to be called "A Better You."

And I began planning this book in earnest, believing that by telling my story, I could reach women everywhere, women who can change their lives, no matter how impossible their circumstances. I also thought I had something helpful to say about what it really took to meet a man a woman could love. Nothing wrong with hanging around a men's clothing department or joining a church—as long as you look good and feel good, as long as the desperation has ended and the confidence has begun, as long as self-esteem is how it all starts.

At the beginning of this chapter, I said that my story had a marvelously happy ending. The happy ending, the real fairy tale, came when I was ready for it. After all those years of struggle, after learning the hard way about the insidious grip of old, destructive patterns and about what it takes to break them, I was all right. Finally, I had discovered that I could live quite satisfactorily without a bad man in my life—although a good one, I still believed, would be awfully nice! Then he arrived.

On a snowy, nasty evening I was preparing for a dinner date with a man I'd met only over the phone. Miserable with a bad cold, the last thing I was in the mood for at the moment was another blind date! Henry Rosenberg arrived at my door. It wasn't love at first sight for either of us. But we did go to dinner, and we talked, and I knew I liked him right away. Two dates later, I realized I had met the man I'd been waiting for all my life—a brilliant, kind, giving, good man, a man of character and integrity. And, best of all, a man who was confident and comfortable with who he was. Henry liked Henry! And by that point in time, Sheila liked Sheila! Before I'd faced my fears and deficiencies, before I'd changed my life, I'm quite certain we would not have found each other.

I moved in with Henry not long after we met. Eight months after that, we were married. And today, a few years down the road, life is better and more joyous than ever. Before Henry, I never understood that term "soul mate"; it sounded to me like just another cliché. Now I know what it means. And I know, also, that it's never too late to find your life's soul mate.

Every woman's story is her own. Every woman's life is different. Perhaps yours has been a mostly happy one, filled with good friends and family and satisfying work. Maybe (and I hope this is the case) you have not experienced anything like the kinds of self-doubt and disasters that I went through on my personal journey. Maybe you've simply reached a point at which you want to make some changes, starting with working on yourself in order to look and feel more attractive.

If there's one message I'd like you take away from my story, it's this: You can do what you want to do. You have the option to change your life, to make today the first day of something new and better.

You have the option to accomplish whatever it is you want, once you begin to believe in the power of change, the power of reimaging.

And any woman can.

PART II
Your Self Analysis

Now we begin with you. First, we will discover what you need to change and why. Later, you will learn how.

Keep in mind that notion of image as the impression you make, in the first few moments, on someone who has never met you before. This is important! Listen to my friend Julia, who began my reimaging program, and you'll see why.

Julia is fifty-five, has been married for twenty-five years, and is the mother of a twenty-one-year-old daughter. She is, in her own words, "very lucky and very blessed." An accomplished musician, Julia teaches classical guitar and piano in a music school and with private students. She's an expert cook, and a relaxed and welcoming hostess to her family's friends. Her husband, Jack, thinks she's terrific.

Julia told me: "I had my thirty-fifth college reunion this year, and my old roommate, Laurie, came in for the occasion and stayed with us for a couple of days. We hadn't seen her in years. Later, Jack said to me that Laurie had aged so much, while I hadn't changed at all! 'You look exactly the same as you always did,' he said."

On Mother's Day Julia received a hand-made card from her daughter, with a "note to bring a lump to your throat," she said. "And to make you feel so proud. At the end of it, my daughter wrote, 'I think you are absolutely brilliant and absolutely beautiful!'"

So what could be the problem with this sunny picture? "I *don't* look the same as I always did," said Julia. "In fact, Laurie looked great! I didn't. I don't look absolutely beautiful. I look like a mess!" She'd been slowly gaining weight over the years, she said, and admitted that climbing a flight of subway stairs got her huffing and puffing. She felt tired from "hauling around thirty-five more pounds than I should." She wore the same kinds of clothes as she always had, "which I must admit are kind of aging hippie-type things, perfectly okay for a guitar instructor, but hardly glamorous."

She had been thinking a lot lately about the future, the next chapter of her life, and her thoughts had been following some new lines: "I want to retire from teaching when Jack retires from his company. And I'd like us to do some traveling, have some adventures, have some romance! I've got a good marriage, but it's also a stodgy, set-in-our-ways marriage." Julia wanted to look better and feel better "just for myself, too. Wearing pants with elastic waists all the time is getting damn depressing!"

Okay, she should lose some weight, she knew. But what else? How did she really look now? How did she want to look? She needed "an overhaul," she said, "a tune-up." But where to start?

The point about my friend's story I want to make to you now: The people who adore Julia, who live with her year in and year out and know the full measure of her worth as a human being, see her through the eyes of love. To them, she's "absolutely beautiful." And yes, she is lucky and blessed to have such love in her life. But Julia was sharp enough to realize that, despite all this, her image was not what it could be or more importantly, what she wanted it to be. She didn't feel great about herself. So she began the process of change, following my steps to analyze what needed to be done to improve the impression she made with her face and body and wardrobe. She was determined not to rest on her family's compliments, and to try to see herself as would someone she'd never met before.

That's a discovery she needed to undertake herself. She started where I did all those years ago—and where you will start now—

with a good, long, hard look in the mirror.

Over the following three chapters, you and I will proceed very methodically through your self analysis. By the end of it, you will have a little notebook filled with thoughts, facts, impressions and other information about your face and hair, your skin, your body. You will have taken the time to listen to your speaking voice, and to consider your posture, your walk, your gestures. You will have considered your wardrobe, and, in all likelihood, done some serious weeding out.

You will have a firm handle on just what needs to be changed. The Program will be underway.

CHAPTER 3

The Mirror Test

Is the mirror your friend? My guess would be no, if you are like most women. The mirror is a welcome friend to only a fortunate few who look and are perfectly pleased by what they see.

For the rest of us, the mirror is a nasty thing! Or it's merely utilitarian, something to use to put on makeup. The typical woman keeps her visits there short: She looks, and she makes a little face. Maybe she squints, maybe she puckers up her lips or sucks in her cheeks—any small, unconscious move that effectively distorts her true vision. Knowingly or not, she's reached the point of scurrying past or diverting her eyes from store windows or any shiny, reflective surface. Even great-looking women do this! I know, because I have seen it again and again when I first begin to work with my clients.

Ellie, a woman I worked with, told me this funny/sad story about herself. "I've become rather good friends with one of my neighbors, Phoebe," she said. "We've gotten in the habit of getting together for a glass of wine and a good, girlfriend-to-girlfriend gab whenever my husband and her boyfriend are out of town on business. And I'm always insisting Phoebe come up to my apartment instead of me going down to hers. Why? Because she has a ceiling-to-floor, wall-to-wall mirror on one wall of her living room where we sit, and I'm trying to avoid that damn mirror at all costs! I can't even enjoy my chardonnay, because I'm forced to look at myself!"

We have those bad habits, formed over years, to break. As

much as possible, we just don't look in the mirror! Or we look, but we don't really see ourselves. We don't really want to see, because it's too discouraging or too painful.

You are about to take a good, hard look.

Starting now, you will accept and even welcome the mirror as your friend. Or you will at least think of it as your main tool toward self-help. I'm not there to have a private, one-on-one consultation, as I do with my clients. All you have is yourself, your mirror, and the choice to either lie (or stretch the truth a little), or to be honest.

I assure you that if all this is going to work, you *must* be ruthlessly objective—a daunting challenge for us all! You may discover aspects of yourself you never quite noticed before, and that make you uncomfortable or even miserable. Perhaps they will even make you more miserable than when you started. Can you handle that? Yes, of course you can! You can because you have embraced your new cause. You are ready to begin the process of change.

The Set-Up

First, find yourself a really good, full-length mirror if you don't already have one, a mirror that reflects your entire body while standing. Situate it in a room with excellent lighting. Find yourself a good hand mirror, a large one, if you don't already have one.

Set aside four separate sessions for the mirror test, ideally on four consecutive days. Analyzing your image is best during daylight, which might mean an early morning session, before heading off to work. If you can't manage a daylight mirror test, make sure your room is well-lighted for an evening session.

Pick a time for each during which you will be uninterrupted, and allow at least thirty minutes—although I would prefer you to conduct your mirror analysis for one hour each time. There's a reason for making this a lengthy, lingering stare: As the minutes pass, you will find yourself sinking deeply into the reflection before you in the glass, avoiding the habitual tendency to glance quickly and then away. You will begin to become genuinely acquainted with the woman in the mirror. You will begin—perhaps only tentatively right now—to embrace her, her shortcomings and her possibilities.

Equip yourself for each session with a spiral bound, blank note pad and a pen or pencil, and perhaps a comforting cup of coffee or tea or a glass of good wine to ease the trauma!

Turn the answering machine off.

Relax, clear your mind.

Sitting or standing in front of the full-length mirror, I'd like you to talk either out loud or in your head to that woman you're looking at in the third person—that is, as "she," an individual separate from your old self—as you answer as objectively as you can the questions I will suggest.

This is critical: View the woman you will be looking at as you would a stranger! We women are great at judging other women. Now it's time to do the same for yourself.

As you look, analyze and talk, make detailed notes. Actually, I would like it if you allow yourself at least fifteen minutes of just looking and studying before you jot down any thoughts. A word of caution: You may be inclined to answer my questions with sugar coating or, to the contrary, with savage harshness. Avoid being too easy on yourself (that old demon, denial) or too hard on yourself (another old demon, self-hatred). Remember, you're not defending or prosecuting the woman in the mirror; you are conducting an inventory, perhaps the first-ever truly thorough and honest analysis of your image.

And when you are finished, you will have on your note pad the blueprint for many of the changes you will soon begin to make.

SESSION ONE

First impressions: Dressed your best

For this session, look as good as you ever look—that means, wear an outfit you consider flattering or appealing, style your hair as you usually do, apply makeup as you usually do. Ask yourself the following questions (and make notes of your answers):

• If you were seeing the woman in the mirror for the first time, what broad adjectives first come to mind to describe her? Would you call her pleasant-looking? Confident? Plain? Angry-looking?

• Do you like looking at her in the mirror? If not, why?

• Would you like her to look like someone else? If so, who and why?

• What one adjective would best describe her makeup? Unobtrusive? Bland? Bright?

• Why does she consider the clothing she has on one of her "good" outfits? It hides her body? It's safe? It's colorful?

• What clothing colors does she think are her "best?" Why? They cheer her up? They go with her skin? What colors does she avoid at all costs? Why?

• Are you comfortable with this woman and like being with her? Can you be alone with her and enjoy her company?

• Do you consider her a secure person? What makes her feel most insecure about herself, or when does she feel that way? With men? Attending a party? In the company of other women?

• Where and when does she feel most comfortable, most herself? At work? In her own home? With her children?

- Would you say other people enjoy being with her?
- Does she consider herself sexy?
- Does she consider herself desirable?
- Does she consider herself intelligent?
- Does she consider herself emotionally well balanced?
- Does she consider herself a success? In her professional life? In her personal life?
- Would a man she's never met before find her attractive? If yes, why? If no, why?
- Does she take care of herself? Eat correctly? Work out?
- How would she like people to describe her? How do people probably describe her now?

SESSION TWO

The unadorned head: Dressed around-the-house comfy

All right, you have allowed yourself a break after that first unflinching look. For session two, wear whatever makes you feel relaxed and comfortable—sweat suits, shorts and T-shirt, your soft and soothing old bathrobe. We'll be ignoring your body for the moment, putting it on the backburner as we concentrate on your image from the neck up.

Wear no makeup. Sit before your full-length mirror, lean in closely, and study that woman's head. List all positive and negative aspects about each area of her face. Take your time. This analysis will require much thought and consideration.

Ask yourself:

- Do you like her face? Enjoy looking at it? Think it's pretty?
- Does she have a "best feature?" Does she do anything to "play it up," show it off, attract the eye to it?

• Does she have a "worst feature?" Anything she's doing in an attempt to downplay or disguise it?

• If she had three magic wishes, what feature would she change first? How would she change it? What's the second feature she would change? The third?

• Tie her hair back or in some other way get it off and away from her face. What is the basic shape of her face? Oval? Round? Long?

• What adjective or adjectives would best describe her hair? Thin? Fine? Thick? Frizzy? Shiny? Dry-looking?

• Does the style of her hair suit the shape of her face?

One by one, study her eyes, nose, lips, teeth and smile.

• What adjective or adjectives best describe each feature? Small eyes widely spaced? Eyes of a pretty color? Prominent nose? Cute nose? Nothing-much nose? Thin lips? Crooked smile? Friendly smile? Gummy smile? Straight teeth? Prominent teeth? Yellowish teeth?

Bring your hand-held mirror to the window or up to the lamp, and take an even closer look.

• What adjective or adjectives best describe her skin? Clear? Porous? Oily? (And yes, skin can still be oily at age sixty!)

• What color tones predominate in her skin? Olive? Pink? A combination of colors, somewhat splotchy? Brownish colorings under the eyes? Bringing her hair down around her face, does the color of her hair do anything nice for her skin?

• How would you describe that woman's neck? Long? Short? Crepey?

Session three

The body, partially covered: Bathing-suited

Before we proceed to The Full Monty—the hardest bit of self-analysis for most of us forty-plus women!—consider your body piecemeal.

Dressed in a swim suit, or in your underwear, looking in your full-length mirror, focus again on the woman you see, and consider these questions:

• What adjective or adjectives best describe her upper-body? Broad-shouldered? Sloping-shouldered? Stooped?

• How would you describe her arms and hands? Firm arms? Flabby? Delicate, long-fingered hands? Workmanlike hands?

• How would you describe her legs? Hippy? Muscular? Shapely ankles? Pouchy knees?

• Does that woman have patches of cellulite, those dimpled fat deposits that can appear not only on thighs, but also on the backs of arms, on the knees and elsewhere?

• Is the skin of her body smooth? Are there small broken veins on her upper body, arms or legs?

Session four

The body, fully revealed: In the nude

Here we are now at your fourth and final mirror test. No clothes, no makeup, the unadorned you. Standing, and using the hand mirror at times, study that woman's body from the front, the side, and the rear, and consider these questions:

• What is her basic body shape? Is she pear-shaped (bigger on the bottom than the top)? Top-heavy (broad-shouldered, narrowing down to thin legs)? Shapely (the hourglass figure, same-sized shoulders and hips and nipped-in waist)? Tall and lanky? Big and round? Small and round? Petite?

• What parts of her body does she like the most? What parts the least? Why?

• Is her body generally well-proportioned?

• Is her body generally toned, or is it starting to head south?

• Again with those three magic wishes, what part of her body would she change first? Second? Third? Larger breasts? Smaller, more defined waist? Slimmer thighs? Longer neck?

• Viewed from the side, does her stomach hang out? Do her breasts sag? Does she stand straight, forming a line from ears to shoulders to hips to knees to ankles?

• Is she overweight? Does she care?

• Are there parts of her body she tries always to camouflage through her choice of clothing?

• Does she find it unpleasant to look at her body?

• How would she feel about a man seeing her naked?

Good for you! I'm guessing the mirror test has not been a pleasure. But if you answered honestly and analyzed objectively, you passed!

Go back over your note book, if you want, and add to, elaborate on, flesh out, think over. Write down your impressions in any style that feels comfortable to you. Some women who have put themselves through the mirror test end up with a series of brief jottings, almost shorthand notations. Some others, I have learned, also draw little sketches for themselves.

And one woman I worked with sat in front of her mirror with her glass of wine and a tape recorder, and had a conversation with herself. You might be amused—and encouraged—to hear a little of what Meredith had to say about her woman in the mirror. Part of that dialogue, which she played for me, went like this:

"Okay, what's your first impression of her? Some adjectives to describe her? Frumpy. Jowly. Slumpy. Sit up straight, Meredith! Much better.

"Something positive to say about her eyes? Well, there are two of them, and they work. Anything else? They're blue. Any particular shade of blue? I don't know...pale blue, I guess. Paul Newman blue. Terrific, she looks like Paul Newman, only not as cute. Would she trade those eyes for another color? No. She likes the color! The eyes could be a little bigger, the eyelashes could be a little more luxurious, but the blue is nice.

"Okay, what about those eyebrows? Definitely need work. When I look at her eyes, the first thing I see are eyebrows. They're not bushy, exactly, but they're...too much, or too shapeless. Are they fixable? I think they should have a curve, but yeah, they're probably fixable. This lady needs tweezers!

"Relax now and look at her forehead. Argh, that I hate! It's flat, actually kind of concave. Maybe she needs bangs? Some way to soften, or let's just call it disguise, the forehead?

"Her nose? Does this woman love her nose? It's the family nose, like the Hanovers, except we're not royal, and all my life I've hated it. But noses are fixed all the time. How can I tell what I'd look like? Remember, we're talking about *her* nose—should she fix it? No, I don't think so. It's a good nose, a no-nonsense nose."

And so it went, Meredith's conversation with Meredith. By the end of her tape, we were both laughing—and Meredith was raring to go with her reimaging. In her notebook she had made the following three lists. You might want to do the same.

Must Change.

Probably Can Be Improved.

Leave Well Enough Alone.

She was ready for The Program.

Put your note pad, that blueprint for great changes to come, away for now. Take a day or so to think over what you observed about your appearance. Sleep on it. Then, consider five final questions:

- Did you truly like the woman you saw in the mirror?
- Did you find pleasure in the way she looks, the way she feels about herself?
- Is she happy with her life?
- Does she want to change her life?
- Why?

Perhaps like my friend, the happily-married Julia, you feel that although a "tune-up" is clearly called for, life is good. Or perhaps, like so many women I have worked with, you have come face to face, literally, with hard truths you have been avoiding for years.

I'd like you to hear one more story, from Helen, a fifty-five-year-old woman who said that taking the mirror test had been a powerful, moving experience for her, filled at the end with tumultuous emotions. After we talked, I asked her if she'd take the time to write down what she'd told me, and she agreed. Here is what Helen wrote:

"I followed your questions, took notes. I wouldn't say that anything I was seeing was a *total* surprise. My body was not in very great shape. I have been gaining weight over the years. I have a perfectly good face, with straight, strong features. But in my 'good' outfit and 'good' makeup, I looked only presentable, at best. My hair seemed faded, and boring. No style really at all. My main makeup for years has been foundation base, to cover up little unevenness in my skin color. I don't do anything with my eyes. There was nothing about 'her,' the woman in the mirror, that was offensive or objectionable. Room for improvement, I thought. Still, who doesn't have room for improvement?

"But something happened, and this was toward the end of session three. I'd already spent by then about three hours all together, looking at the woman in the mirror. And I was suddenly looking past the features, the hair, the skin. I was looking deep inside, and tears came to my eyes. I was seeing back, back to myself when I was about twenty-four, twenty-five.

"I was always very proud of my hair, for one thing, always got compliments on it. I've always had a good head of hair, and in those days I really cared for it. I wore it in a style that was sort of a soft, swingy flip. And I'd learned that the best way to achieve this was to wash my hair at night, dry it completely, then set it in a few big loopy pin curls and sleep on that. If the hair was too damp, it came out too curly the next day. So, no matter what time of night—maybe I was getting in from a date at 2 a.m.—I'd go through my hair routine. I might have been dead on my feet tired, but I did this. Just so I'd look great the next day.

"I washed my hair brush and combs once a week. Shaved my legs every other day. Nobody knew much about waxing back then! And I'd rub lotion into my legs. Once a week I lathered up my feet with Vaseline and wore socks to bed. Kept my legs and my feet soft and delicate. I invested in a very good scale, and once a month, I'd weigh myself. Only once a month—I never wanted to turn into one of those people obsessed with weight. If I'd added a couple of pounds, I started walking more, cutting down on certain foods. All kinds of things I did. I paid attention to myself.

"When you're young, you have so much hope! So many things seem possible. But I also had a good, 'pull up your socks and get going' attitude. If something wasn't right, I could make it better.

"When I was looking at the woman in the mirror, and tears were coming down, I wondered what had happened to all that. What happened to that person? I had a sense that in some strange way I almost didn't exist anymore. I was divorced almost fifteen years ago. My son, just off to college now, and my daughter, halfway through high school, are my life. If I get depressed these days, I give myself a little talking to, remind myself of the good things in my life—my great kids, a rewarding job. Remind myself of a couple of friends who died too young and I should be thankful just to be alive. Tell myself I have no complaints.

"But staring in the mirror, I missed that self I used to be. No, not to be twenty-five again, but to have some of that feeling of hope, possibilities, options, gumption. To be that woman who took pains with her appearance, who tended to herself in those little ways. To be that woman who thought it was *important* to tend to herself. I'd lost that 'pull up your socks' attitude—if it's not right, do what you have to do to fix it. And there are things about my life that aren't right, that should be better. When I was answering the question of where I felt most comfortable, I decided it was getting into bed at night, wearing my baggy old nightgown, reading my book, not having to see anybody for the rest of the day—escaping. That's not how I want my life to be!

"And Sheila, I ended up where you did in front of your mirror. I realized the woman in the mirror could change. I realized I was wrong, off track, and absolutely mistaken to accept from myself less than the best of myself. I owed myself something better."

That was two years ago. I wish you could see Helen today. She is an absolutely marvelous looking woman, but more than that, she radiates joy, confidence and energy. She decided to never let it be too late. She accepted that okay is not good enough.

I want you to do the same.

CHAPTER 4

Added Reflections (maybe
with a little help from a friend)

Brutal objectivity in front of the mirror will take you far. After the mirror test you may have a pretty clear idea of what you want your reimaged self to look like—new hair, less-flabby body, more becoming makeup. Remember, however, that reimaging has to do with the total package. That means how you speak, how you stand, how you walk into a room, what your body language says about you all have to be taken into account. It's what I call learning how to make a charming presentation of self.

Rena, an enormously successful businesswoman in her early forties, came to me with the story that I hear so often. She had reached a very high rank not only in her particular corporation but in her whole field. She met men all the time in the course of her work, she had business dinners with men and traveled to corporate events with men. They clearly admired her skills and expertise—and not one of them ever had suggested the two of them get together for something other than business. Once again, here was a woman who hadn't had a date in years, who woke up one morning and wondered if she'd let all her chances for a personal life go by the board. She started asking herself what she was doing wrong.

I asked her, "What is it that you want?" And she answered, "I want to be a desirable woman." So Rena and I got started on her reimaging. She needed to do body work (losing weight, toning up) and face work (a great new hairstyle, among other things). She needed to add to her all-business wardrobe some "desirable" clothes. She went about all this with her customary diligence, focus and discipline, and, about eight months later, she looked fantastic. Gorgeous! And nothing happened.

Rena looked lovely but presented herself badly. For one thing, she talked in a masculine, all-business manner, with "yep," "nope," and very forceful, let's-get-this-deal-done comments and responses. A friend arranged an introduction to two men, each of whom called her on the phone, talked to her for a while, and then ended the conversation without suggesting they meet. From her friend, Rena got some feedback: Her two potential dates just didn't like the way she sounded! Her voice and manner of speaking turned them off.

She had to go back to the drawing board, and make some adjustments in her presentation of self.

This is what you and I will consider now, as we take your "before" picture one step further.

You'll do a little candid camera work, looking at some photos of you in various situations—and as we know, the camera doesn't lie.

A tape recorder will come in handy for listening to the sound of your own voice, and analyzing whether it is as appealing as it might be.

Also, if you possibly can, ask for a little help from a friend. The careful, considered and honest suggestions of another woman can round out your analysis and uncover further aspects of your image that could do with fixing, the aspects you can't see very clearly on your own. Remember, you want to use every tool at your disposal, and the tool you'll put to work here is someone I'm calling your confidante, a wise and considerate woman who'll lead the way to a more subtle level of analysis.

CHOOSING YOUR HELPFUL CONFIDANTE

It may make you uncomfortable to approach someone and ask her to give you an honest critique of your image. While *you* may suspect what your flaws are, you certainly don't enjoy the prospect of hearing that they're obvious to everyone else as well!

You'll think of asking a person you're close to, and your rationale will be how well that individual knows you. Who better qualified, you might assume, than your sister, or your best girl-friend, to give you the real lowdown and tell you what needs changing? Fine. Ask, and listen to what she has to say.

But I really believe your very close friend, your mother or your sister aren't your best bets. These people are too involved; they care about preserving your relationship, and they'll worry about hurting your feelings. Or, there's a lot of history between the two of you that may color her comments and observations. She may be kind and compassionate, but she may not be entirely truthful, or she may genuinely not see those quirks or characteristics you possess that really could do with your reimaging attentions.

Instead, give some serious thought to asking a colleague from work, or a neighbor in your building. Or you may want to ask the distant relative you typically see only on holiday family get-togethers, but have always liked for her warmth and candor. The person you seek should be the woman who always seems well-turned out, attractive and groomed. She should have good taste, and should be someone you think has a good image. She should seem to draw people to her in an effortless and positive way. Maybe it's someone you've admired for years and recognized as a woman of great personal style, and whose opinion you've valued. Someone who makes you think, "Boy, I don't know how she does it, but she always looks damn good!"

When you find your candidate, tell her what you're doing and how you would like her help: "I'm reimaging myself, and I could use some advice. I'd like to ask you some questions about the impression I give off, and I'm going to rely on your keen, objective eye. I want you to be absolutely honest, and that will be the most beneficial and kindest thing you can do for me."

This individual might be disarmed by your request. At the same time, she should be quite complimented too, since you are saying, in essence, "I trust you, I think you look wonderful and confident, I'd like to become as chic as you!" Make the whole matter as pleasant for her as possible by inviting her out for lunch (you will pay, of course) or even better, to your home for a glass of wine some evening.

WHAT TO ASK YOUR HELPFUL CONFIDANTE

Your first key questions: "How do you see me? How would you describe the overall image I present? If you were meeting me for the first time, what would come to mind?"

When Georgia, a woman beginning her reimaging, asked these questions of her confidante, she heard a mouthful! Georgia described that meeting: "I admire this woman enormously. We've worked in the same company for some time, although not closely together. But I've always noticed the way she moves through the halls, the way she answers the phone. Her clothes are simple, but seem designed for her body. People seem to like talking to her. Her manner is both friendly and slightly aloof.

"And that's the way she was with me. She said, 'Georgia, this is wonderful, what you're doing for yourself! I admire you for it. And I'm happy to help you in any way I can.' Then, in the course of the next half hour, I learned that, in her opinion, I gave the impression of being thoughtful and intelligent, and also somewhat tentative when I talked. I learned that in her opinion, my eyeglasses were all wrong for me and covered up my pretty eyes. I learned that I gave the impression of wanting to hide my body, because I covered it up with very loose clothing. I learned that I gave an impression of being somewhat unapproachable, because I didn't smile often. I learned that I was missing a great opportunity to show off my natural coloring by wearing shades of peach and burnt orange."

This woman had a lot to tell her, Georgia said, and was able to do so in a warm, encouraging and supportive manner. If your chosen confidante is not so immediately forthcoming, ask specific questions concerning your appearance.

For example, ask: "Do you think my clothing suits me? Would you call it too conservative? Would you say it's feminine?"

"Do you think I'm ready for plastic surgery?"

"I've always been self-conscious about my smile and my sort of crooked teeth. Is this a very significant part of my image, something you notice right away when you talk to me? Or am I making too much of the whole thing?"

Ask her whatever you'd like to know more about.

THE WAY YOU REALLY SOUND

You can do this with your confidante, or just with a friend who's come over to visit. Put a blank tape in a portable cassette player, press "record"—and then forget about it as you and your friend talk. Pretend it's not there. I'd suggest you also take a tape recorder reading when several guests are in your home for a dinner or cocktails or whatever.

Another time, record your side of a phone call. Have your little cassette player loaded and ready to go, press "record" and let the machine pick up your part of the conversation.

At some quiet point, listen to these tapes, and pay attention to how you really sound. Decide what image your voice suggests, and if you can call it a pretty part of the package. Does it contribute to a charming presentation of self?

Many of my clients confess to feeling unhappy at the sounds of their own voices when they hear themselves on tape (and are delighted to learn, as you will later, simple ways to improve them). One woman I worked with was quite surprised at what she heard. "I have a kind of monotone voice that sounds tired, or maybe blasé," she said. "Also, I say 'Uh-huh' or 'Mmmm' all the time, background noise that's unattractive."

THE ALL-TELLING SNAPSHOT

We might call this the mirror test, Part Two.

The next time you're in a gathering of friends or family, bring along one of those easy-to-use disposable cameras, and ask your friend or sister or another guest to please take a bunch of snapshots of you in the course of the afternoon or evening. Tell her you don't want to be "posed," you don't want to be warned to "say cheese and smile!" Explain that you're just trying to come up with some ideas about how your appearance might be improved, and you'd like some candid photos.

Develop these pictures and study them carefully. Perhaps they will hold no surprises for you. Or perhaps you'll learn a cold, hard truth or two about your *real* appearance, something you hadn't noticed during the mirror test. Pat, a woman doing The Program, said this: "I was shocked to see that I have no neck! Unless I'm holding my head high, putting my shoulders back, which I guess I was doing all through the mirror analysis, my chin disappears into my chest. I'm fatter and softer in the neck than I ever imagined. And this made me look a whole lot older than I am." It gave her some ideas about working on her posture, and possibly losing some weight as well.

Go back to your notebook, if necessary, and add there observations about your face, body or clothes that the candid camera has brought to light.

Is your jaw line a little more jowly than you realized?

Is the tummy a bit flabbier?

Does your haircut look flattering from the front but not so flattering in profile?

THE SILENT LANGUAGE: A MOVEMENT ANALYSIS

If you have a video recorder (or can borrow one), you have in your possession an indispensable tool for seeing how others see you in action. Ask your confidante to film you as you enter a room, as you sit, as you stand and carry on a conversation.

Study this film later, and look for body language that needs fixing:

Do you appear vaguely angry or upset when you walk into a new space? Do you hang your head, look around nervously?

Do you frown a lot when you're talking?

Do you make eye contact with the person you're talking to?

Do you sit gracefully?

Do you sit in a slouchy manner?

Do you "talk with your hands," gesture a great deal as you speak? Considering those movements as objectively as you can, do they strike you as appealing, feminine, or lively? Or do they seem distracting and excessive?

A woman I worked with had the opportunity to observe herself "in action" when her brother left a camcorder running during the course of a long afternoon, a celebratory luncheon for their parent's sixtieth wedding anniversary. What she immediately noticed when looking at this tape later was her body:

"Plain and simple, I just look fat! I look a whole lot heavier than I knew. You can't really tell this about yourself, I think, unless you watch yourself moving around, getting up and down from chairs, see yourself from the back. I know I'm a little over-weight, of course. But my clothes were less of a camouflage, I guess, or less becoming than I believed. This was news."

Jot all your observations in your notebook, that blueprint for the changes to come.

CHAPTER 5

Clothes and Stuff: Separating the Good, the Bad and the Ugly

Virtually every woman I have worked with has let her clothing closet take on a life of its own. She has her reasons for hanging on to all that stuff: This outfit cost a lot of money. This doesn't fit at the moment but when I lose weight it will again. That one is too youthful but maybe my daughter will want to wear it sometime. Or maybe: This is how I've always dressed, and change is scary.

Sound familiar?

Perhaps you, like most of us, have read an article about closet clutter, vowed to make improvements, and then abandoned the task. You may be familiar with the advice: Arrange jackets, slacks, dresses and blouses in separate areas, according to color; buy special bins for storing sweaters; get stacking racks for your shoes, and so on. I'm all in favor of organizational strategies and hardware—if you possess a large wardrobe of varied clothes that all fit well and all look modern and smart, and you are blessed with lots of storage space.

Probably, you don't have such a wardrobe and you aren't blessed with all that space. If you've decided it's really time to reimage your looks and your life, I'm guessing that you have not so much a large, workable wardrobe, as a pile of clothes, only a handful of which you actually wear these days. Your closet space may be limited, or given over in large part to other possessions that need to be put *somewhere*. So suggestions to organize by item, color and so on may be simply unworkable for you, or downright discouraging. You're not ready for organizing strategies and hardware until you know what you've really got, and analyze what you really should keep or not.

In this chapter, I want to suggest a simple approach, geared to a simple goal: Every piece of clothing hanging in your closet on any given day will be wearable and will look good on you. If achieving that goal means that at the conclusion of this part of your self analysis you have only three such items left, fine. We will build from there! Three great outfits are infinitely preferable to the dispiriting sight of a rack full of stuff you can't or don't wear. You know that already! You've read that a hundred times! Now it's time to act on what you know.

When I work one-on-one with a client, I go to her home, and we tackle her clothing situation together. We separate the summer, winter and year-round items that are hanging in there. Many, many women, I've discovered, don't follow this simple, seemingly obvious practice. And there may be perfectly understandable reasons for not organizing by seasons: Space is limited, that's the main one. Or, you had planned to put away the light-weight stuff early in September, you never got around to it, and here it is January, so why bother anymore?

I have my client try on every piece of clothing she owns, check for fit, look at herself in the mirror, and ask herself: Am I going to feel great when I go out the door in this? Many times, the woman I'm working with will say, Well, the answer is no, and why do I still have this anyway?

We separate out everything that looks awful and old. Separate date clothes (if there are any) or evening clothes from day clothes. Separate out items that don't look great at the moment, but that she loves, or really wants to keep, and that can be adjusted.

I can't be with you in your bedroom, but in this chapter I'm going to do the next best thing—give you some pointers, and encouragement, to help you figure out what to keep, what to store, what to repair, and what to give away or throw away. Again, when you can open up your closet or your drawers and pull out anything in there and know it works, it not only simplifies your whole life, it does wonderful things for your head!

Before we start, let me tell you about Beverly, and what her closet revealed at the start of her reimaging. Beverly conducted her clothes-sorting and weeding out on her own, and told me how it went:

"I live in a very lovely, very old apartment building. Back in the late-twenties when it was built, apparently builders didn't pay a lot of attention to clothes closets. My bedroom has one closet that's not very wide, but for some reason is very deep and high. Some years ago I installed a rod across the back, so I have two rods to hang things on, although you can only reach the clothes in the back by shoving aside everything up front. Up above there are several shelves that go up to the ceiling, which I can't get to without standing on a ladder. Basically, it's a ridiculous, inconvenient, inadequate closet.

"So, emptying everything out of there as you advised me to was a miserable, messy, depressing experience! And it went downhill from there! Here's some of the stuff that I piled on my bed and on the chair and the floor:

"Fifteen blazers or jackets, wool and lightweight. This is what I wear to work every day. They all look pretty much the same— boxy, unstructured, covering the hips and with shoulder pads. Seven of them are black or gray. Then there were various pairs of slacks—again, my usual work outfit. On the back rod, the Siberia of the closet, were pants, blouses and a bunch of skirts that are too small now. I hardly ever wear skirts anymore, but it seems I've kept a lot of them—from a couple of old minis to ankle-length. There were some skirts from my ethnic phases, long, gauzy and with bright patterns. Most of the stuff in the back is the thin wear, from when I didn't weigh so much.

"I have three outfits for evening, each one of which I bought on the run, at the last minute, because I needed something for a fancy wedding or whatever. And I never did really like any single one of them and also I paid too much for them. Also, they're fat wear.

"Strange, bargain purchases—a long white cotton shirt from Mexico with embroidered baskets and flowers on the top, which I thought would be cute to sleep in, and which I've never used once. A turquoise suede bomber jacket kind of thing, which I remember looked garish as soon as I got it home. Also never worn. A blouse with sequins, on sale, that I thought would dress up this fairly decent black, crepe pants suit I have. A denim, muumuu kind of dress, also on sale, that I thought I'd be living in for doing chores in the neighborhood and so on, and that looks like a tent. More random stuff of that sort.

"From up on the shelves I got down handbags and an insane assortment of stuff. Shoeboxes full of family photographs. Empty boxes that I use for wrapping up Christmas presents. A large canvas tote bag full of small canvas tote bags with logos on them that I guess I thought would come in handy someday.

"Shoes on the closet floor. My shoes, actually, were the one bright spot. I actually like them and wear them.

"Is this depressing, or what?"

I'm telling you Beverly's sad saga, because this is the starting point for many women, and perhaps it will be for you. I want you to know that if the thought of analyzing your wardrobe is just too grim to contemplate, you have much company. The time is now, however—to go through all that stuff, and to be clear-eyed, objective and even ruthless about what stays and what goes. When I work with a client, I utilize everything of hers that we possibly can. Often, an item of clothing just doesn't fit properly, and can be adjusted. Or the impulse purchase she's never worn would look great with the right accessories.

You had the courage and the determination to take the mirror test. You can deal with your clothes!

Starting Small: Drawers First

Closets do tend to be overwhelming, so get your analysis started by tackling your drawers. Empty them on your bed, one by one, and check out everything you find. Make the following decisions:

• Pretty, feminine underwear is nice to have, but not essential at this point in your reimaging. Fresh underwear—that is, panties and bras that are not torn in places or have droopy elastic—*is* essential. You don't need more than seven pair of panties and two or three bras to get from laundry day to laundry day. Weed out the excess or the tired. Buy a new set of inexpensive underthings tomorrow, if you have to. You've got to feel good from the inside out.

• Check sweaters, tee-shirts, sweat suits and the like for holes, tears and stains. If the item is old, tired, permanently stained or doesn't fit, and has a hole or a tear, toss it. If you come across that really nice wool pullover that you forgot you had, and you remember you haven't worn it because it was pulling apart at the shoulder seam and you couldn't find the little packet of repair thread that came with it initially, put it aside for possible resurrection. Maybe the tailor at your local drycleaners can fix it.

Beverly made a bold move at this stage: "I have one drawer that's full of old tee-shirts. They go back years. Most of them have things printed on them, and I only wear them around the house. I remembered all of a sudden reading an article about an older woman who was moving out of her house and into an apartment, and she said she was getting rid of everything, just taking with her two chairs and twelve white tee-shirts. I thought that was so neat! So I decided now, out with all these shirts! I'm keeping two old, soft Mickey Mouse shirts that I like to sleep in, that's all. And I'm going to buy a couple of nice, well-made, white tees for the rest of the time."

So many women have that "grubby" little wardrobe, the old tees and shorts and whatever that they wear while cleaning or sleeping or repainting the moldings, that have been washed two hundred times and that of course they'd never wear elsewhere but can't imagine doing without. Hold on to a couple of these useful items if you have them, but don't keep a drawerful of them. Especially if you've been depressed, feeling lonely or just not very great about yourself, it's too easy to slip into the old, worn, faded and comfy as soon as you walk in the house. Much better for your reimaging cause to wear something inexpensive but pretty and fresh, even if no one sees you but you.

• Throw out any single items that are supposed to be half of a pair. A bunch of lone socks that don't match are a downer.

• Throw out pantyhose with the beginning run or with the heels that are all pilly. Foraging around in a pile of old pantyhose looking for a decent one is not a part of your new style.

• Like many women, you may have a stack of scarves in your drawer. Give these your clear-eyed attention. One client I worked with had twenty or more of the small, twelve-inch silk squares that were once popular knotted tightly around the neck. She hadn't actually worn them this way (or any way) in years, and admitted that she never liked that look on her in the first place. She had a couple of other scarves—one, a long, flowy silk print that had been a gift; the other, a bargain purchase of her own, a long, white, heavy silk crepe with fringe on the ends—that were unusual and interesting, and that she'd never used. We decided the little squares should go, and the other two should get a life (with a new outfit or two in the future).

Don't hold on to a "good" silk scarf (just because it has a name brand) if it's faded or unraveled in the hem. You don't need it.

Okay, you've cleared out and organized your smaller stuff. You are feeling, I hope, revitalized and energized. You are steeled now to move on to the bigger stuff.

TACKLING THE CLOSET

Time for the major job.

As you already know, I'd like you to empty the closet. Everything out! Set aside a full day for this, if you possibly can. As you go through each item in there, one by one, ask yourself some questions: Are my clothes primarily...

• Someone else's idea? (What the fashion magazines said was in?)

• Things I bought only because the price was right?

• Things I bought on impulse? Or at the last minute, because I never seem to be ready with the right outfit for a particular occasion?

• A lot of the same thing? (You always think it can never hurt to have one more black blazer?)

• All over the color map? Or all solid neutrals?

• All clothes I wear to work?

• All big and loose with no defined waistline in sight?

• Things I bought because I thought they were right for the job I had then, and I haven't worked in that field for years?

Obtain a general idea, in other words, of what has motivated your clothes buying or accumulating. You'll probably come away with some useful thoughts of what you should stop doing, or of some gaping holes in your wardrobe.

Try on everything, one by one. Look in your mirror; ask yourself: Does this really fit me properly? Do I love this? Do I look great in this?

MAKING PILES

The great weeding-out begins. Separate your clothes into separate piles, as follows:

1) Items I will toss.

Probably there will not be as much in your closet as there was in your drawers that should be pitched. But again, any items that are badly, irreparably faded, discolored or stained, or that are shabby or torn beyond repair, are of no use to anyone, much less you.

Slacks that are old and have been worn a lot start to sag in the rear. They will never un-sag and revert to their original shape. Get rid of them.

2) Items I will give away.

If you live in a large city or good-sized community, almost certainly there is a thrift shop in your vicinity or a church that conducts annual clothing drives. Pass along to these worthy outlets items of clothing that you will not wear in the future. These should be in decent condition, of course, and they may include clothes that don't fit, can't be adjusted, and you don't much care for anyway; clothes that you sort of like but realize look dated, too juvenile, or less than great; clothes that you liked once, but have to admit do not become you at this stage of the game (maybe the ethnic-style skirts that looked cute on your twenty-year-old self); clothes that you haven't worn in a year or more and don't know why you bought in the first place.

I recommend, also, that you cast a stern eye on the multiples (like Beverly with her fifteen blazers, seven of them black) and consider whether it really does you much good to keep them all. Maybe you'll want to hold on to them. Or maybe you can do very nicely with fewer of the same thing, and thus you will free up your closet and your mind by weeding out.

Add to your giveaway pile the odd pieces (think of Beverly again, with her denim muumuu and other "random stuff") that you never use, or that you realized long ago were a mistake, and that you've been keeping in there simply because they're there. Rid yourself of them now.

If there's a piece of clothing you think your daughter or your niece might like some day, give it to her now and tell her to keep it for the future. Get it in her room or her house, and out of your closet.

3) Items I don't wear, or haven't worn in ages, but maybe can re-invent.

These are hard decisions to make on your own. Maybe these questions will help:

Is there a dress that's nice, well-fitting, good color, but you don't like the puffy sleeves?

A skirt that's passable, but might be great if it was four inches shorter?

A two-piece suit that's severe, drab and boring, but the jacket might come to life if it was paired with something very different, like a print skirt?

A decent-looking dress that might be turned into a fantastic strapless dress? (Yes, we are going to talk strapless in the next section!)

Use your imagination, and see if you have a few items that can be re-cycled, perhaps with the help of a local tailor.

4) Items that don't fit, today.

Remember the goal of your closet analysis—you want to be able to reach in there and pull out a piece of clothing that looks great on you, right now. That means it needs to fit, right now.

When Beverly weeded through the Siberia section of her closet, that back rod that held her "thin wear," she found some items she really loved and wanted to hold on to—a couple of well-made, lined wool skirts; a couple of tailored dresses. All size ten. Beverly was size fourteen. Beverly was determined to lose weight, to bring her dress size down again; it was central, in her mind, to a successful reimaging. And she wanted to keep those couple of skirts and dresses, and wear them again one day.

More power to her, I say. And to you, if you share her goal and her determination. But get that stuff out of the closet! It is **not** inspirational or encouraging or motivating to look at some items of clothing that you can't fit into, every time you go into your closet. Do what Beverly did: Pack those things up in a little carton (or fold them up in a drawer you don't use), and store them somewhere.

5) Items that are not in season.

Do set aside the spring and summer stuff if it's winter now, and put them elsewhere. Pack those things up in a little carton if you don't have a spare closet and store them under your bed, if necessary. You can buy inexpensive, long and flat boxes designed for just this purpose. You will feel more in control of your appearance, more elegant, if you keep your closet's contents seasonal.

Reloading the closet

Now you're ready to put things back.

Try to arrange your edited wardrobe by size and style. Group blouses all together, dresses all together, jackets all together, day clothes all together and evening or dressy clothes (if you have any) all together. I'm guessing you'll be very pleased by the sight of this. Said Beverly: "When I got everything back in the closet, there was air space between the hangers. For some reason this thrilled me! The closet looked sleeker, and it made me feel sleeker."

Do something about your shoes, if they live on the closet floor. Buy one of those inexpensive shoe organizers for the floor or to hang on the door. Buy one of those bins or baskets now, for belts or small handbags.

Try to turn your clothes closet into a welcoming little place! I love the idea of giving it a fresh coat of paint in a cheerful color or wallpapering it, but I just throw that out as an aside. We don't want to turn this into the never-ending job! If at all possible, don't use that area for storing on the shelves or the floor those boxes of family photos you mean to organize someday, or the Christmas ornaments, or other odds and ends that we all seem to carry through our lives. Stick those things anywhere else.

Getting ready to head out into your day should be a pleasure. Together, you and I are now going to figure out how to make it more so.

PART III
Changing Your Looks: The Program

We have the "what" agreed upon. You know what you want to change about your face, your body, your wardrobe, the sound of your voice or the look of your walk. Now we get down to the hard work of "how" you will make the changes you know should be made.

First, a word about money. Some of the women I reimage have lots of it. No problem for them the head-to-toe makeover that might include an entire new wardrobe, plastic surgery or other costly improvements and on-going maintenance. Let me lay my cards on the table here and give you some specifics. In the Introduction, I told you about one of my reimaging clients, a woman who sold her business for millions and then went to work on herself. She was serious, dead serious, about what she wanted, which was to turn herself into a gorgeous-looking, feminine-looking, fantastic female who'd attract men.

She initially purchased, with my guidance, a seventy-seven-piece, brand new fall and winter wardrobe. She's since acquired an equally glorious spring and summer wardrobe. She underwent a series of laser treatments to improve the appearance of her hairline, which was low on her forehead, and had surgery to raise her gums and give her a prettier smile.

Although her major reimaging (including losing about twenty-five pounds) has been accomplished, she has a professional facial every other week, a pedicure every other week, a manicure once a week. Twice a week she goes to a salon for a blow-dry on her hair. When she's preparing for an evening out, she has a professional makeup application. Once a week she gets a waxing to remove unwanted hair on her body. Every three months she has the hair on her head un-frizzed.

Is all this costly? You bet. Does all that servicing help to keep her looking great? Absolutely. And does all this mean you have to drop a ton of money on your reimaging? Not at all.

Most of the women I work with do *not* have lots of money, not by a long shot. Most are very conscious of budget considerations. I am imagining you may have a fairly limited budget too, and limited time as well. You *still* have an enormous number of options available to you and you *still* can work small miracles with The Program.

That said, I will add this: Break the budget a bit! Splurge! Let go!

This is all about the rest of your life, and this is time to spend the very most that you can. Eliminate, for the time being, some of the small indulgences you now enjoy but that have nothing to do with the reimaged you. Keep on getting manicures if that's one of your indulgences—lovely hands and nails are a must. But cut back on restaurant meals, take-out gourmet food, maybe even this year's vacation trip.

My point is: Keep your mind on the cause, sacrifice now and devote as big a chunk of your finances to the program as you can. You won't regret it.

In this section, we are going to proceed methodically through the steps in your reimaging—your hair, your face, your body, your clothes, and what I called your presentation (working on some of those clues you might have picked up with a little help from a friend). You'll find that the suggestions relating to these matters are not elaborate or exhaustive or full of every last little detail. There's a reason for that.

I said at the start of this book that almost all of my clients already *know* a great deal about what it takes to look good. You probably do too. Any intelligent, reasonably informed woman can hardly have missed reading or hearing all this good advice—how to lose weight, what an eyelid lift can do for you, why it's advisable to moisturize the skin every night and apply sun block every morning, and so on. The women's magazines are full of it; news reports constantly update us on the latest developments regarding nutrition or cosmetic surgery or workouts. Go to your local bookstore, and you'll have no trouble browsing through any number of books devoted exclusively to skin care or exercise or simple-but-chic dressing.

However, like so many women I've worked with you have been neglecting what you know, or you concluded a long time ago that these "beauty tips" are aimed squarely at the twenty-something or the thirty-something audience. Or, more typically, you have been failing to pull the pieces together and work at them diligently with the particular goal of reimaging yourself in mind.

So, in the following chapters we are not going to re-invent the wheel. I'm assuming first, that you already have a lot of useful information stored in your head; second, that you are now *really* ready, mentally, to start acting on what you know as well as on the advice I'll give you; and third, that you are remembering the cause.

What I want to offer you in the chapters to come are some specific tips, reminders, warnings, and options that I know are pertinent to the older woman. What I want to tell you now is this: All the changes outlined in the next section are things you can do.

You cannot inject yourself with self-esteem. You cannot decide that starting next week, you'll have courage and confidence. But you *can* decide that starting next week (or better yet, starting today) you'll begin the changes we'll talk about. The steps are clear and concrete. They are foolproof. They work for anyone and everyone. They do not require any intrinsic feelings of security and power. They just require doing—and you can do it!

Pull out your notebook again, look over all the observations you wrote down during your mirror test, and now let's see what you'll do next.

CHAPTER 6

Your Hair

Did you conclude after that long, thoughtful study of your face and head that you have little to lose and possibly much to gain by considering a new hair style and/or new color?

Perhaps, like many over-forty women, your self analysis revealed a conservative head of hair—neat and low-maintenance, but generally unremarkable. Louisa, a woman who completed the program, had noted this: "Hair basically the same for the last twenty years, a short cut with a few bangs. Mousy color. Self-coloring to touch up gray. Looks kind of lanky and skimpy. I never had what you'd call a great head of hair, even as a kid. So my thought, I guess, has always been the less said about it, the less noticeable about it, the better!" Louisa was more than ready for some new thoughts.

"New" hair—a different color, a different style—is the biggest, quickest confidence booster you can find. The look of your hair can make or break you, accentuate your beauty or kill it. And yet her hair is what usually makes a woman crazy! Aside from the look of her thighs, her hair is what she most hates.

At the same time, I also have come to realize that changing her hair is one of the scariest moves for the over-forty woman. It's a funny thing: When she was younger, she may have thought nothing of trying out one look or another. She had a breezy, "it's only hair, it'll grow out" attitude about the whole matter. Somewhere along the years, she lost her courage when it comes to experimentation, and the hair has been "basically the same" for a long, long time. She's in a rut, afraid to change.

Does this sound like you? Do not be afraid! Today may be just the day for you to consider a serious change in your color and style. However, get ready to splurge. This is one of the times I really do urge you to open up the purse and spend more than you think you should, at a good hair salon and with a good colorist. Ask around or read around, and get recommendations. Decide to go for the best, one that a friend or a woman you know who always looks great swears by.

I also believe you should do a trial run on the place you choose. This takes a bit of nerve—many good salons, or the highly-touted or very busy ones, aren't terribly comfortable to walk into. A bunch of sleek, slim, cool-looking individuals are gliding around, ready (you think) to cast judgment on your poor head. There's nothing wrong with stopping in, talking to the stylist, admitting to your trepidation, getting a feel for the person who may become such a critical cog in your reimaging program. If you don't feel right about him or her, or suspect you'll be getting a polite (or not-so-polite) rush-through with nobody paying much attention to your real needs, look elsewhere! Find the place that's right for you.

When you take the plunge, I think you may be stunned at just how much confidence a new, stylish cut and perhaps a new color will give you.

Let's consider what might be right for you.

BEST CUTS FOR DIFFERENT-SHAPED FACES

The following general suggestions may be helpful as you mull over what hair style will best suit the shape of your face and head. But I'd also suggest that you pick up a couple of the latest fashion magazines on the newsstand, look through them and find some cuts you think would be flattering on you. Bring that clipping to your hair person, tell him or her this is what you had in mind—if the stylist is a good one, he or she will give you an honest opinion (yes, a good possibility, or no, not really best for your hair and face.)

Go even one better than that: See if there's a wig store in your city, visit it with a friend who'll offer her candid opinion, and try on various heads of hair. Get a fresh idea or two.

From your mirror test—the part during which you pulled your hair out of the way and tried to analyze the shape of your face and any of its especially noticeable characteristics—you will probably have come up with one or more of the following conclusions:

• *If your face is oval*

Lucky you. It's the classic shape that no style looks really wrong on.

• *If your face is round*

The prettiest style for a basically round, no-discernible-cheekbones type of face is a soft look with some hair feathered forward onto the cheeks. Such a cut will slim your face and make it appear more oval.

• *If your face is long and thin*

Probably you will not want to go too short or too long—either length will tend to make your face look even longer and thinner. A medium-length, chin-level cut might be most appealing.

• *If your face is square*

A chin-level cut is often best for this face shape, too. Avoid a center part, the all-around blunt cut, or anything too sharp and linear.

• *If your forehead is high and pronounced*

Try cutting a few wispy bangs. You'll be amazed at how this simple change will soften your face, and make you look younger too.

• *If you have a long, prominent jaw*

Avoid a super-short cut or an upswept style. They won't be flattering.

LONG HAIR...SHOULD YOU?

Yes, men like long hair, and some (few) women can wear it long even in their fifties and sixties—if they are "good with hair," clever about styling, perhaps pulling it back or up into twists and letting wisps fall around the face. Katherine, fifty-two, is an example. She has a head of very thick and wavy, lustrous pale auburn hair with no gray, which she usually winds into a loose, high bun or coil and secures with an interesting decorative comb or clip. Sometimes at outdoor, casual affairs, she lets this glorious mane float around her face and shoulders. She's a knockout.

Generally speaking, long hair is not for you, unless you have what Katharine has—a lot of healthy, shiny hair of a good color. If you are not so blessed, short is definitely better.

Short hair can take years off a woman's face. I know: The shorter I've cut my hair, the more compliments on my youthful appearance I've received. (One of the most stylish women I know is over-seventy, and has a Joan of Arc crop cut; no hair on her head is longer than an inch!) But remember that for most women, layering hair and making it "move" is terribly important for a truly appealing, feminine look, and this absolutely can be accomplished with a short cut. The helmet-head—over-sprayed, fixed, lacquered—looks old, old, old.

BEST COLORS FOR DIFFERENT SKIN TONES

Again, I hope that after studying your unmade-up skin in a good light you came away with a notion of your basic skin color. Perhaps it wasn't what you always thought it was—skin tone changes, often pales, over the years. Or perhaps you hadn't really looked at your face without makeup, in a hand mirror, in daylight, ever before. In addition, you brought your hair down around your face, and looked hard at what the color of your hair was doing for the color of your skin—and maybe you decided, not much! Or, it looked perfectly okay, but you realized you were tired of the same old hair.

Time for a color change! Here are some very general tips to consider as you think about what that might be:

• *If you have pale-to-white skin*

Chances are you can adopt any new color and it will look fine.

• *If you have pink or ruddy skin*

Ashy, somewhat neutral or hard-to-define colors will probably be most attractive with your pinky skin. Extreme colors—like a vivid red or a very yellow blond—will be considerably less attractive.

• *If you have yellowish skin*

Dark tones are best—a deep auburn or a chestnut brown might nicely balance out the sallow tints in your skin.

• *If you have olive skin*

Dark hair is best for the olive-skinned woman as well.

FOUR BIG COLOR MISTAKES NOT TO MAKE

Changing your hair color can be wonderful, exciting—but don't try to get there yourself! At the beginning of my own reimaging—in fact, on the very first day that I started to change my life—I bought a coloring kit at the drugstore, spent an hour in the bathroom and emerged with a head of Nordic blonde, as I described to you earlier. I also said back in that chapter that I absolutely do not recommend self-coloring like this, even though many new (and improved) home-coloring products are on the market. Inevitably you'll come out with all-over, one-color hair, and for most women that's harsh, aging, and unflattering. And a cheap look. And anything but natural. Young, gorgeous women can get away with the obviously colored head of hair. Most of us older women can't.

For any kind of coloring, I do urge the splurge, and the professional job. Find a beauty salon that specializes in coloring, or that has a colorist on the staff—an individual who's an expert. Get up your courage and talk to this person a bit before taking the plunge: If you don't like the color after you're finished, what can be done? How much maintenance is going to be required to keep it looking good?

Then remember these four common mistakes that older women so frequently make, and avoid them:

• *The one-tone blonde*

If you have light brown or brunette hair and you've decided on a blonde tone— either lightening your natural "mousy" color or even trying a dramatically pale, champagne hue—highlighting your natural color is the best way to start. Tone-on-tone is the prettiest look, and a good colorist will have a couple of ways to achieve this. If you have substantial gray in your basically brown hair, you may need to have a base color applied before highlighting is possibly. This is somewhat expensive, but worth a try.

Highlighting will last for two or three months before you need a touchup. If you're contemplating a dramatically lightened shade, so that new hair growing in will look very much darker, accept the fact that you must schedule and pay for those touchups! The Meg Ryans of the world can get away with the dark-roots look; you can't.

•*The red redhead*

I have seen only a very few redheads I think look great, unless it's a woman's natural color. The red dye once used has been banned in the United States as a cancer-causing substance—all to the good. However, the various tones of orange and auburn typically in use today can produce, unfortunately, an extremely artificial result. If you are determined to go red, never do it yourself! Find the best colorist you can, and discuss with this individual how to achieve a soft auburn or perhaps reddish blonde tone.

•*The inky brunette*

Stay away from hair that's too dark or black—those shades will add years to your appearance. If your naturally brunette hair looks dull or flat, try taking the color up a notch to a chestnut brown, and see the difference that can make. Highlighting for brunettes can be wonderful, and add instant life to your hair. Again, get thee to a good colorist!

•*The love-me-love my gray*

"I am what I am, gray hair and all, and if anybody doesn't like it, too bad!" If such is your line of thought, fine...keep your gray hair. But very few men find will it attractive.

There are a few fabulous-looking gray-headed ladies out

there, including a couple of very busy older models. In my opinion, the only woman who can stay beautifully gray is the one who has almost everything else going for her—elegant, well-defined features, including beautiful eyes, great cheekbones, and a splendid smile; a well-proportioned, fit body; good clothes; and thick, healthy hair to start with.

DOING IT YOURSELF

I've given you my lecture about going to a good salon for your coloring. That's because a professional will in all likelihood achieve a more subtle, becoming effect than you can manage on your own, and because only a skilled individual can perform proper highlighting—and highlighting is what looks prettiest on many women. If your budget really won't allow the professional job, however, and you've decided to go for do-it-yourself color, spend some time studying the products available to you:

• *permanent color*

This is good if you have a lot of gray you want to cover. The color, as "permanent" implies, stays in until you cut your hair, so it's wise to be pretty certain you're pleased with the color you're choosing. If the color is very different from your natural shade or if you're going to all-brown from all-gray, be prepared to touch up the roots on a regular basis as new hair grows in, probably about once every one-to-two months.

• *temporary color*

Some shampoos on the market offer temporary color, which will last through a few shampoos and slowly wash out. Temporary color (not effective if you have a whole head of gray hair you want to change) might be nice to try if you want to check out the effect of a slight or subtle color change but you're not ready for a major commitment.

- *semi permanent color*

Like the temporary dyes, semi permanent color won't do much for gray hair that wants to be something else. And like those, you'll get a rather subtle change. If you're basically content with your brown hair but wish it would look less mousy and more lively, look for a semi permanent kit close to your natural shade—you can get some shine and life, without going way different. Semi permanent color washes out over a dozen or so shampoos.

Too thin: what to do

Almost one in three women by age fifty has thinning hair. And too many of those women conclude, "Cut it short, get it permed, and it'll look fuller."

The short-and-permed look is often the instant-old-lady look! Certainly, shorter is preferable to longer if your hair has thinned out over the years. But consider what else you might do to improve its appearance.

Should you consider extensions, those added pieces that give you the look of a great big head of hair? Extensions are a complicated business, and are created in various ways (gluing, weaving, clipping on). Probably this is a bit more expensive, time-consuming, and high style than you want to consider. For a special occasion, however, it's good to know that such things exist.

A woman who has genetic hair thinning—it runs in the females of the family—might actually be able to stop the loss and have a good percentage of hair grow back, by following certain diet plans and hormone and/or drug therapies. If you're interested in giving this a try, ask your doctor; he or she should be able to put you in touch with a specialist who can offer good advice, which might be a dermatologist or an endocrinologist.

But really, an excellent, layered cut can do wonders for your thinning-out hair by giving it lift, movement and the appearance of more volume than you ever dreamed of. Do experiment with the cut, before deciding on the perm and risking that helmet-head look.

TOO FRIZZY: WHAT TO DO

If you have frizzy hair and have longed for straight hair, it can be yours quite easily these days. Again, I'd advise against the do-it-yourself approach, although kits are readily available. Straightening the hair requires the use of strong chemicals, and you want to put yourself in experienced hands (the same holds true if you want a perm.) These modern treatments are extremely effective, as long as your hair is not over-bleached or damaged. Find a qualified salon with a stylist experienced in straightening—it's called anti-curl or relaxing—and explain your wishes.

Ask this wonder worker for suggestions on how to care for your newly unfrizzed head. You'll probably have to get used to moisturizing your hair regularly and often, and some products are especially recommended for straightened hair.

What you have been calling frizzy, however, might actually turn out to be charmingly wavy and bouncy, with—again—an excellent cut. And also, with regular trimming of the ends.

GET INTO PRODUCTS!

My friend Alexandra vowed, as she approached her forty-fifth birthday, to reimage her looks and change her life. Alexandra has a twenty-one-year-old daughter, soon to graduate from college. Alexandra said this: "When Molly was home from school on a long break, I noticed her beauty products, all the stuff that instantly took up half the space on the bathroom sink and on her bureaus. I was amazed. For the hair alone, there were various mousses, gels, muds, lotions. There were things to mold, shape, thicken... volumize, a word I didn't even know was a word! Products to vitamize and therapize!

"As far as my own hair goes, I have two things I use—a bottle of shampoo and a bottle of conditioner. I mentioned this to Molly, and she said, 'Mom, it's time for you to get into products! I'm taking you shopping.'"

Mother and daughter spent an hour in their local cosmetics and beauty supplies shop, and Alexandra left with about fifty dollars worth of "new stuff for my hair. It was so much fun! I got home and felt like a teenager, experimenting with all these delightful items."

There's a message I'd like you to take to heart. It's not my intention to urge you to spend money on hair care products. Splurging on the good, professional cut and the good, professional coloring I think is essential. After that, maybe your old favorite shampoo and conditioner are all you really need. Shampoos, you should know, are all pretty much the same. The inexpensive variety will do for your hair exactly what the pricey one will do, which is clean it.

But maybe this is your time to consider new products, check out the stores and find out what's available. Buy a set of rollers—the Velcro ones are pain free and easy to use. Experiment with "new stuff!" Many of us haven't done that in years, and there is an amazing array of new things out there. A bagful of these items need not set you back a bundle, either. Many of the inexpensive brands contain the same ingredients as do the high-ticket versions. Poke around!

You might have some fantastic results. Besides, you'll have fun. And I told you, you're going to start loving all this.

We started with your hair first, because I do believe that restyling and, perhaps, re-coloring can produce an instantly greater-looking you. It's really the quickest, simplest way to get an enormous psychological "up." If you need a jump start—visible proof that good things are underway—this can do it for you. A great-looking head of hair will give you the biggest bang for your buck, and it's a wonderful motivator to keep on going on with your reimaging cause.

CHAPTER 7

Your Face and Skin

Your mirror test and photo analysis of your face may have left you somewhere along the continuum from "room for improvement" to "radical overhaul called for!" Maybe you came up with some very specific thoughts: "I should probably find a way to emphasize my eyes more, because they're nice." "Can I do something about my chicken lips?"

Or maybe you weren't thrilled with what you saw, but have only general notions of how to proceed. One woman said this: "When I was in my thirties, makeup did wonders for me. I had a real 'before' and 'after' look. With no makeup on, I looked perfectly okay but nothing great. Then I'd put on my face, and wow—great! Now I just have a 'before' and a 'before' look. Even in my 'good makeup,' I never have that feeling of wow, I look great! I just look like an aging woman who's put on some makeup."

Let us talk about options!

What follows is anything but an exhaustive listing of products and treatments and so on. I simply want to point you in some directions, suggest some possibilities, remind you of a few things, and issue a couple of warnings.

IF YOUR MAKEUP NEEDS REIMAGING

The over-forty women I work with seem to have one of two attitudes concerning makeup. One type says something like this, what I heard from Jackie: "I used to fool around with makeup when I was in college and in my early twenties. But I finally figured out what looked good on me, and I've stuck with that." She stuck with it too long, I told her—the lime eye shadow that she thought was good with her blue-green eyes and the chalky lipstick weren't horrible. But they were making her look dated, or at least, not her best. Jackie had actually started to come around to the same conclusion during her mirror test.

The other type says: "I don't use makeup. Never have. Maybe just a little pressed powder and lip gloss sometimes." Some women can get away with the minimal-to-non-existent. Usually, however, the woman who doesn't wear makeup because she "never has" is missing out on a good bet.

If you too decided it's time to re-think this whole matter of makeup, I'd urge you, first, to experiment a little! If typically you buy a fashion magazine once a decade, buy several now. Look at the colors that are currently in fashion; maybe they're not for you by a long shot, but you need some fresh ideas. Then spend a little and try out a product or two that you think might produce an appealing result.

Do *not*, I suggest, let one of the "cosmeticians" at your local department store go to work on your face with their line of paints and potions. In my experience, most of these individuals have no idea what they're doing, and hope only to sell you as many products as they can. Inevitably, you'll end up looking "done," in a most heavy-handed way.

Don't let them brow-beat you into buying stuff. One of my clients was searching for an oil-free, lightweight foundation base—she'd never used a foundation before. On three different days she went to three different counters in a large department store, and was persuaded to buy three different products, each of which was too heavy, too greasy and the wrong color for her skin. She had been intimidated by her shopping; she was annoyed with herself and discouraged by this first venturing-out into the world of cosmetics. Don't be put off by salespeople. Sometimes you can get samples of particular products. Don't be afraid to ask for them.

I do think, however, that if your budget can possibly stand it, it might benefit you tremendously to make one visit to a professional makeup artist. Ask around among women you know, stop in at one of the spa-type salons, or check the style pages of your local paper or magazine, and come up with a name. You can pick up some wonderful tips on colors that might look fabulous on you and that you would never have dreamed of, and on how to apply all that stuff. This individual also can give you a lesson in eyebrow shaping (more about eyebrows below).

Keep in mind, at all times, where and how you can so easily go wrong, especially if you haven't been much of a makeup maven for a long time.

I'd like you to know about:

EIGHT BIG MAKEUP MISTAKES: WHAT THE OVER-FORTY WOMAN SHOULDN'T DO

- *Too little of a good thing*

A lot of women who don't feel truly comfortable, as one woman said to me, "putting a lot of gunk on my face," or may have never used foundation or mascara, decide they'll give it a try. All to the good. Then they get timid and tentative about experimenting. Or they've used nothing but pressed powder and lipstick, and go about reimaging their makeup by trying new shades of those two items, but nothing else. Or a woman will try eye shadow, but put only a little dab in the middle of her lid.

They get nervous about "putting on a face!" But your over-forty face might really appear a great deal brighter, livelier and prettier with more makeup than you've traditionally used.

- *Too much of a good thing*

The opposite of too little! Over-applying makeup when she's over-forty will age a woman faster than any almost anything else. Too much foundation, eyeliner or, most of all, powder is a big mistake. Powder will get into your little wrinklets and creases, and make them stand out, and add years to your look.

Occasionally when I was modeling for a fashion shoot years ago, the makeup person layered on coats and coats of powder—supposedly to keep my makeup in place and my face un-shiny. I've looked at some of those old photos lately, and realized I appeared ten years older than I was. Scary!

Use a light, translucent powder, and use it sparingly. Any piece of makeup that's applied with a heavy hand will not help you. Gorgeous twenty-somethings may get away with a lot of shadow, for example, and the very bold, dramatically-colored eyelid. Most of us older women will seem only clownish doing the same. Accentuate your eyes with a warm, pale shadow. It can be in a shade of blue or green, or in one of the lovely beiges, mauves or light, pinkish browns. This will accomplish the trick as naturally as possible. A well-known makeup artist who works with many celebrities says, "Don't wear colors that do not occur in nature." I think that's a pretty good rule of thumb.

Go gently with the under-eye concealer. If you don't already use this and realized at your mirror test that those brownish patches under your eyes are more noticeable than you thought, do experiment with a tube of concealer. But apply with a light hand! Nothing looks worse than an attempt to disguise under-eye bagginess with a heavy slash of concealer; you'll just look like you have overly made-up bags.

Foundation should be as close to your own skin color as you can find, and lightweight.

• *Too trendy*

Yes, do check out the fashion magazines and learn a little about the fabulous array of makeup products available to us all, and what the models are doing these days, and what *the* colors for next spring will be. *Don't* go trendy—say, with navy blue mascara— because it's the in thing. Again, trendiness sits better on the twenty-somethings.

• *The runaway lip line*

Heavily-lined lips are a huge no-no! Why this is I'm not exactly sure, but all sorts of women seem to be walking around with dark colors outlining lighter colors on their lips. Super model Naomi Campbell does it, and on her it looks great. On you, it won't.

Lip lining is actually most beneficial to the older woman. Perhaps your mirror told you that your lips have lost a little of their natural definition, or have those tiny lines sprouting out from the upper edge. With a liner—either a pencil or a brush— you can define and build out your lips slightly, and make them appear a bit more voluptuous. But fill in your entire lip with the same color. Apply a little translucent powder over all, then another dab of lipstick.

• *The deep, dark, red lip*

Bright red lipstick is usually a mistake, especially if your lips are on the thin side. Too garish, too clown-like, and invariably aging, as is a frosted lip color. Soft, muted shades really are best; bright but soft tones in coral or apricot are pretty too. But do use some color on your mouth. Even if you have full, well-shaped lips—which you've been content just to dab with a touch of lip balm—a little color is going to make them look more appealing.

• *The deep, dark, black line above the eye*

I like eyeliner. I think it can do great things for any pair of eyes, opening them up and emphasizing their color. The women I work with, however, typically don't use eyeliner at all or are stuck in the rut they've been in for years, painting on that ebony black line.

Try a eyeliner pencil (much easier to use than the brush and liquid liner variety) in a dark gray, dark brown or taupe, and dot in a line along the outer half of your lid, close to the lashes. Then soften the line with your finger.

• *The misplaced blush*

Blush is something you should definitely put on your "must try" list, if you don't already use it. If you know you're looking a little pale and anemic, blush will give you an instant pick-me-up. But again, not too heavy—and not in the wrong place.

Brush it on in soft strokes from the center of your cheek and out towards the top of your ears, covering your cheekbones. If you have fabulously high and defined cheekbones, try a little blush *under* the cheekbones, to highlight this attractive feature. I like to apply a touch of blush to my forehead and the tip of my chin, too, to add a little glow.

• *A makeup for all seasons*

This is the one thing almost every single woman I've worked with does: Whatever she's using (foundation, powder, lipstick, eye shadow, whatever), she uses *always*— day and night, winter and spring, summer and fall. And I call this a mistake, because the same stuff doesn't always do the same job. For evenings out, you're wise to go for a little bolder or more exciting color. In summers, your wintry powder will look awful. You really do need at least a small variety of products.

A FACE TO WEAR OUT AT NIGHT

So what might you do for an evening out? You'll use your normal foundation and powder, but you might take some other things up a notch. Consider:

- a slightly darker powder under the cheekbones to gave your face a slimmer-appearing contour (something you don't want to wear in daylight)?
- a bronzing powder brushed on your cheeks, to add a little light to your skin?
- a bronzy or silvery shadow for your eyelids, again for a bit of gleam?
- a top coat of a silvery or gold gloss over your regular lipstick?

Do start thinking about playing up your reimaged self in one of these ways for a date or a night out, of which there will be some in your future!

EVERY WOMAN'S MOST IMPORTANT FEATURE

It is—are you ready?—the eyebrow. I would call this the single biggest mistake almost all my clients make—letting those eyebrows do whatever they want! I am ferocious on the subject of eyebrows, and I believe—I *know*—that most women have no idea what a big, big role they play in enhancing the face. Your eyebrows, all by themselves, powerfully affect your facial expression. They can give you, literally, the appearance of looking happy or sad, angry, masculine, or just plain plain. They are critical to your reimaging program, and I say that without even knowing what you look like. Eyebrows can make or break you! Clean them up. Train them. Maybe give them a little lift and an arch.

Eyebrows are wild creatures by nature; they have to be tamed. If your brows are bushy and growing every which way, get in the habit of brushing them into shape (set aside a fresh toothbrush for just this purpose) when you just step out of the shower and the hairs are damp. You can mold them into place over night with a little Vaseline, getting them used to where they should be.

Immediately, go and buy a good pair of tweezers, and spend a few moments in the morning, in good light, plucking out the strays and shaping, one hair at a time.

If your face is long, your brow can be on the straight side. For most facial shapes, a slight arch, highest at the center of your eyes, lifts the face and gives it a cheerier, more welcoming look. The common wisdom says: Hold a pencil vertically across the center of your eye, to see where the brow arch should appear.

Consider whether a little, light plucking under your eyebrows might help define their shape in this attractive way. At the least, don't let stray hairs straggle out at the ends.

IF YOUR SKIN NEEDS REIMAGING: THE FOUR MUSTS (AND ONE NICE MAYBE)

Makeup, of course, can improve your looks dramatically. And like a great haircut, it's good for an instant high—and a whole lot of encouragement to keep forging ahead with the program. Next we'll look at what you should be doing to renew and repair the skin itself. Actually, it's almost a given that we over-forty women need skin reimaging, or at least, some attention must be paid to our skin!

Aging first makes itself most visible in the skin. Perhaps for you, as for so many of my clients, facial skin aging is not so much a matter of lots of wrinkles and sags, but rather a dulling of tone. Perhaps after your mirror test some of the adjectives you thought of to describe your skin were "faded," "pale," "dried-out."

You've already heard tons of information about protecting and treating your skin. In the department store beauty section or your drugstore or cosmetics shop, you'll find just as many products as there are for hair. Will some of these items improve the look of your skin? Absolutely. Can you have some fun trying things out? Of course—and I do want you to have some good, feminine fun with all this! Should you expect miracles? You know better than that. You can't eliminate wrinkles or bags with lotions or creams. But there's a lot you can do to have prettier skin.

Do drink lots of water. Do get an adequate amount of sleep. Do consume a diet of healthful foods, such as fresh fruits and vegetables and grains. Those are the basic rules for keeping *all* of you looking and feeling good.

Besides that, this is what you should remember about:

• *protecting your skin*

Stay out of the sun and wear sun block, with an SPF15 or higher reading, summer and winter. Put sun block on the backs of your hands, too. The sun's rays will wrinkle up and age your skin faster than anything, and can cause more serious damage as well. It's easier than ever to get protection, because many moisturizers, and even some foundations, contain blockers.

Stay out of the sun as much as possible. When you are exposed to sun, wear a hat. Every time you let the sun hit your unprotected face, you're destroying cells that cannot be replaced.

• *cleaning*

What's most important to remember about cleaning your skin

is simply to keep your skin clean. That means, of course, never going to bed without removing everything you've had on your face all day (you knew that). Most women I work with are pretty good about this necessity, and also have found through trial and error what works for them. That might be a product designed to remove makeup and clean the skin; it might be good old soap and water.

Whatever you use, be gentle. Pulling and tugging will stretch that delicate facial skin.

• *moisturizing*

Most of us need a good moisturizer, to keep skin soft and not feeling and looking dry. Professional makeup artists often like to dab a light moisturizer on to clean skin, let that sink in for a while, then apply makeup when it's dried. If your skin is on the dry side, that's a good bet for you.

Go heavier at night and slather on a good moisturizer in upward strokes all over your face and neck.

• *getting rid of dead cells*

Skin really can appear fresher, pinker and younger when the top layer of flaky, old cells is sloughed off. A good—gentle!—rub with a washcloth will accomplish this ex-foliating. A mask— which you apply over your face, let dry, and then peel off or wash off—is fun to use every so often. And the relatively new alpha-hydroxy and beta-hydroxy acids, found in creams and lotions, can brighten the appearance of your skin if you use them religiously over time.

When it comes to all these skin-care products, don't drop a ton of money. For great-looking hair, I think you have to splurge (as you know). For this stuff, you don't. You can make yourself a little crazy these days reading all the ads for lotions, creams and whatnot that promise all manner of results. We now have available (so a recent ad tells us) an imported cream that will positively "re-invent" the appearance of your skin; a tiny pot of this can be yours for $450. Please!

Great-looking skin has a lot to do with the genes (if your mother and grandmother had it, lucky you) and a lot to do with protecting, cleaning, moisturizing and a little ex-foliating. You can't do anything about your genes; for the rest of it, inexpensive products you pick up at the drugstore are probably going to do exactly the same job as the pricey stuff.

• *the beauty salon facial*

This isn't a must, but I'd urge you to try a professional facial in a good salon, if you haven't had one before. You will get a deep cleansing and moisturizing, your pores will be ridded of all that clogging debris, you may have a mask and a toner applied, you may receive a light massage. Maybe you'll love it so much, and see such great results, that you will decide to budget into your life the every-other-month facial. All to the good, I say.

However, this word of warning: A professional facial puts your skin through a pretty rigorous workout. The best time to schedule one is probably not right before you have a big evening out or any social engagement. Your skin may initially look worse (blotchy and red) rather than better. Actually, if you come away looking really red and blotchy and have skin eruptions over the next few days, that particular treatment was too harsh for your skin.

Do find a reputable salon—ask friends what they recommend. Explain to the individual who'll be "doing" you what you know about your skin and its sensitivity. Some of the products these places use may be too irritating for you, and you can avoid possible problems by keeping the lines of communication open.

IF YOU NEED HEAVY-DUTY REIMAGING

When Diana studied her face in a good light she found herself focusing on her neck and on the skin of her upper chest, around the breastbones. She didn't like what she saw: "I had lots of little mole-y things on the sides of my neck and on my chest. I guess I was always vaguely aware of these, but I never realized before how many of them there were and how unattractive they were. I thought of barnacles on the side of a ship. I thought I really should get those barnacles scraped off!"

Diana went to a dermatologist, and learned that her mole-y things were called papilloma, that they do often appear as we get older, and that they could indeed be "scraped off" without much difficulty.

Removing those little harmless bumps that really are not pretty and that detract from your attractiveness if you're wearing anything but a turtleneck is just one of the things a dermatologist can do for you. We are in the age of the new dermatology, and what a boon that is! Among the many strictly cosmetic services these specialists can provide are:

• laser hair removal, a process to check out if you have fuzzy cheeks, and other laser treatments to improve the surface texture of the skin (they can also eradicate bulging leg veins).

• silicone injections to fill in wrinkles and plump up lips.

• prescribed Retin-A creams to minimize fine facial lines.

• Botox injections, which also smooth facial lines like forehead wrinkles and those vertical frown lines on the insides of the eyebrows.

• implants to puff up thin lips.

• chemical peels, to give the skin a deep ex-foliating and get rid of small scars.

• bleaching and other treatments for age spots.

All these modern, non-surgical wonders, which are added to

and improved almost by the month, are yours to investigate if you are determined to take your facial reimaging up a notch, if your budget can stand the strain, and if you find for yourself the very best dermatologist in your area. In the Appendix, my own favorite dermatologist, Dr. Howard Sobel, will provide you with some "what you need to know" basics about these various procedures, and I do urge you to read what he has to say and to think about whether this is a route you should consider.

Ten years after I had my face lift (more about that below), I began to see signs of aging once again—lines on my forehead, wrinkles around the eyes and lips. In my business, it's critical that I look my best, and so I considered if it was time for further surgery. Instead, at my dermatologist's suggestion, I elected to receive Botox injections to deal with the forehead lines (Botox can greatly improve a saggy neck, as well) and silicone injections in the cheeks and around the lips. The result was nothing short of miraculous.

In my experience, these procedures are worth every penny (and they are not cheap) if you want to avoid plastic surgery. Botox injections need to be repeated every few months. Silicone lasts forever (and if it's done to decrease fine lines around the mouth, it will also build up and fill out the lips in a way that looks soft and natural). *However,* if you cannot find or afford the very best expert in your area, don't do it! All these procedures do have possible complications, such as, in particular cases, infection, scarring, mottling of the skin, eyelid droopiness or scabbing. You must work with a qualified, experienced specialist. In the Appendix, my experts address these issues more fully.

GOING WHOLE HOG: PLASTIC SURGERY

I believe every woman should feel the best she can about herself. And I believe you should do whatever it takes to get there. If plastic surgery will help you get a better face, it's not really a lot different than going to a psychiatrist to help you get a better head. But you *must* do your homework first, and thoroughly research the doctors you are considering. I learned that lesson the hard way.

Years ago when I was still modeling, I started to focus a lot on my sagging eyelids, the fine lines around my eyes, and the pouches forming around the sides of my mouth. So I took the plunge and had a face lift. The problem was, my face didn't lift. To the contrary, I suffered through a botched job that left me with holes (yes, holes) in one side of my face, muscle and nerve damage, and months of misery before further, corrective surgery began to repair the damage. I had been foolish. I tried to save money on my facelift and ended up almost losing my face! So above all, what I want to say to you is this: Go to the best plastic surgeon you can find. Borrow the money if you have to. Or if you can't, then don't do it at all! If you decide on surgery, accept the need for a major financial splurge.

This individual should be available and willing to discuss with you at length, before you agree to the procedure, exactly what he will be doing, what you can expect to experience during the operation and as you recover, and what follow-up care will be required.

At the end of this book, one of the experts I have consulted will offer you some overall advice about the types of surgery available. If you're ready to go whole hog, check it out.

THE POWER OF A SMILE

Many a man has fallen in love with a woman's smile. Actually, what a man notices first about a woman's face are her mouth and her eyes (I have this on good authority). You can improve the line of your lips, and make them appear a teeny bit fuller, by putting on lipstick as I mentioned above. And you can achieve dramatically more voluptuous lips by one of those procedures you'll get from a dermatologist. But pretty lips aren't going to be much of an asset if your teeth aren't white, straight and proportioned to your mouth. I know in my own work that I can do everything for a client, but if she opens her mouth to reveal yellowish or greenish or tannish teeth, the case is closed! Bad-looking teeth are a turnoff!

Fortunately for us all, dentists these days can do much more than fill in cavities or cap a chipped tooth. If your teeth are not terribly attractive, they can be whitened, straightened, veneered, bonded and in several other ways made to look quite handsome. Please do read what Dr. Michael Kraus, a cosmetic dentist, has to say in the Appendix about the possibilities available to you.

YOUR BEST FEATURE

Do you have one? We all know if we do or not. A woman I worked with told me she had never elected to get pierced ears, because her ears were perfectly formed, and when she was younger there had been a boyfriend or two who liked to nibble on her exquisite lobes. (Yes!) Another woman remarked proudly on the fact that buying the eyeglasses she needed for reading was sometimes a challenge because her eyelashes were extraordinarily long and full, and batted up against the lenses.

It's wonderful to have a "best feature." And to be pleased with oneself about it. One thing I want to say is this, however: Play it up softly, subtly. Especially when it comes to eyes, many women seem to go too far in the wrong direction. A woman I know has lovely and remarkable eyes, of a pale, true gray color. In case nobody noticed, apparently, she chooses to emphasize this unusual feature by wearing a lot of the same shade gray in her clothes, and by applying—always—a lot of gray eye shadow on her lids and a lot of black mascara. The effect actually diminishes her naturally beautiful feature.

Sometimes you can make too much of a good thing.

CHAPTER 8

Your Body

Men prefer slim women. I have received confirmation of this irritating though unsurprising fact from the several dozen currently unattached older men I interviewed for this book—quite a few of whom were far from trim and taut themselves, it should be noted.

Women prefer *themselves* slim. Although virtually every one of my clients has been dissatisfied with and wished to alter some aspect of her body shape, I have rarely heard any one moan that she was "too thin."

So let's just get that basic truth out on the table. Slim is better than fat.

And let us take a moment to get angry once again about the unfairness of the social world, in which a man can be fat and flabby and still get a woman.

Then let's get down to work!

In this chapter, we'll consider your body, as it is and as it might be. Open your notepad to the observations you made during your mirror test, sessions three and four—when you studied your body first partially clothed and then in the nude. Perhaps, as for most women, these were the most painful aspects of your self analysis. Perhaps, also, after taking a long, hard look at your naked self you decided to get serious about losing weight and toning up your body. Good, good, good! I applaud that decision. Even a *few* fewer pounds can mean a very big improvement to your image.

But ridding yourself of those few fewer pounds—or of many pounds, if you are significantly overweight—will not be easy. This is really the most grueling segment of your reimaging. Getting a new hairstyle and color may have been traumatic, but it didn't call for much effort on your part. You simply had to get yourself to the salon and sit in the chair, and somebody else did the work—and the payoff was immediate. Improving the appearance of your skin by religious moisturizing and by making yourself more skilled and informed about makeup wasn't that difficult to do either. Opting for more serious face work, through plastic surgery or other procedures, may be a *really* traumatic move, but again, someone else did or will do the job for you. Now you're on your own.

Nobody can lose weight for you. Nobody else can make the day-after-day decisions that are necessary if you are seriously determined to achieve a slimmer, more attractive body shape. This is your job, and yours alone! It is no quick fix; it takes time, perhaps a lot of time.

And in the same breath, I want to say to you that *nothing* will make you feel better about yourself (not even that fabulous new hairstyle) than knowing that your body is as lithe and lovely as it can be. Really, it changes everything. You will look younger, you will move more gracefully. You will be able to cross your legs and drape one over the other in that appealingly feminine and sexy manner. Your clothes will hang on your body in the way they were designed to hang. You will have more energy. You will have more courage!

As you get started on reimaging your body, what should you know? What should you remember?

IF YOU INTEND TO LOSE WEIGHT

It takes relentless determination—no big surprise to you. You probably also have already read three dozen articles and one dozen books about how to do it. Everybody and her sister, it seems, has tried or is trying to take off the pounds.

The U.S. Government issued a major statement recently about the whole matter of weight loss, and here are a few startling facts that were offered:

The first diet book was published in 1863. (Goes back a long, long way, this concern with fat.)

There are currently 15,400 diet books listed on Amazon.Com.

The diet industry in the United States is a thirty-three billion dollar (*billion!*) business.

Forty-five percent of women are "on a diet" at any one time.

Sobering thoughts, are they not? But the whole matter of losing weight is really a whole lot simpler than we often make it out to be. Here's what that government report went on to say:

• Fancy, elaborately structured diet plans or weight-loss foods—including all the costly, prepared, pre-packaged products, menus and meals—aren't necessary, and sometimes even a bad idea. They may work for a while, they may get the pounds down, but they won't do anything terribly good for you in the long run. That's because to maintain the loss you must change the way you eat all the time, not just the way you eat while you're "on the plan."

• Calories do count. But what matters is the relation of calories taken in to calories spent out. Eat a lot and move around a lot and maybe you won't gain weight. Eat a lot and *don't* move around a lot, and you surely will gain weight. For most reasonably active women, 1500 calories taken in daily will lead to weight loss.

• Cut down on fatty foods, like steaks and burgers, fries and chips, and eat more fruits, vegetables and grains, and you're on the right path.

I very much like the idea of keeping the matter of *how* to lose weight simple. Yes, it takes time, determination, effort, etc., etc.— but *how* to do it isn't that mysterious. Most doctors, dieticians, and nutritionists agree on a number of basic rules, a set of guidelines that are virtually guaranteed to work for the vast majority of people. We'll review those below, but first, you may be interested in what I've heard from several women I have worked with.

Carla, a woman who said she knows (like most of us) that the weight is creeping on when her skirts feel tight and the waists of things don't close, uses a "foolproof" approach: "I eliminate all the white foods for a while. No bread, rice, pasta, potatoes, milk. A few weeks of this does the trick every time. It's a fail-safe plan."

Maggie told me: "The only way I can drop weight is if I suffer. Total denial of everything I really enjoy eating! I'll have a little bowl of cereal in the morning, and I measure this out, with a half banana and skim milk. Steamed veggies for lunch. A miniscule piece of plain chicken or fish for dinner. This is the equivalent of wearing a hair shirt or beating yourself on the back with birch branches or something. I have to have that feeling of denial and virtuousness. If I have a couple of chocolate chip cookies in the middle of the morning, the rest of the day is shot. I have to start over the next day with the virtuous thing."

A lot of women have their fail-safe plans. And a lot of them go the all-or-nothing route. Such attacks certainly do work, and there's nothing wrong with them for the woman who wants to take off a few pounds quickly or the woman who needs a jump start—the psychological boost that comes from seeing fast results. When you're in for the long haul, however—when you have a lot of weight to lose and you're determined to keep it off—a more balanced approach is the only way that's healthful and the only way, really, that works.

Denying yourself a whole range of foods or "suffering" through with foods you don't enjoy will make you crazy! And you can't keep it up! Human nature isn't like that, and life is too short anyway.

GENERAL GUIDELINES FOR TAKING IT OFF

If you have read any of the better (most reasonable, most scientifically supported) of those 15,400 diet books that can be ours for the asking, you will have learned the following:

• *Accept the fact that losing weight takes time.*

By following a good, healthful diet, you should expect to lose no more than two pounds a week. Typically, you'll lose more when you first start changing the way you eat; then things slow down. Think about that. If you're looking to take off forty or fifty pounds or more, you're going to have to keep at it for a while.

• *As much as possible, prepare your own meals, using fresh ingredients.*

Said Emma, a client who got serious about losing weight: "I'm thinking of an ad on television showing a woman—beautifully though simply dressed—singing an aria while she lovingly, sensuously grates parmesan cheese into a baking dish. There are a bunch of gorgeous red tomatoes and greens and stuff on her gorgeous counter. I love that ad, not because of what it's trying to sell me, and certainly not because I have a kitchen like that! I love it because of something it reminds me about the whole business of cooking dinner. We should try to enjoy the process, we should be thankful that we have so much fresh food to cook with, we should make the whole thing a labor of love. It's a better way to think about food than just as something to get on the table and chow down." I like her way of thinking.

When you prepare your own meals, using fresh products, you also have more control over what goes in them.

• *As much as possible, eliminate prepared, processed foods from your shopping and eating.*

Canned and many frozen foods, including those diet meals, contain a lot of sugar and/or a lot of salt. You don't need those.

• *Eat according to the major food groups.*

Most of us have seen that pyramid-shaped picture of the different food groups, which suggests what we should be eating the least of (top of the pyramid) and the most of (moving on down). Healthful diets include taking in something from the whole range of foods on a daily basis, in roughly the following proportions: Have some protein (meat, fish, cheese, eggs), somewhat more carbohydrates (potatoes, bread, rice, cereal) and even more fruits and vegetables.

You need some butter or oil in your diet. You do *not* need anything to be fried or heavily sauced or otherwise loaded down with perhaps tasty but calorie-heavy preparations.

• *Eat smaller portions.*

A seriously obese pop star underwent surgery to reduce the size of her stomach: From a normal stomach (which is about as big as one or one-and-a-half fists), she went to a stomach the size of a thumb, which obviously could not hold much food. She lost a significant amount of weight.

Surgical re-sectioning is drastic and dangerous, and I'm hardly suggesting it's something you should consider even for a split second. But do think for a moment about that image of the normal, fist-sized stomach, and how small that really is. Think about it when you load up your plate. You don't really need a lot of food at any one time to fill your stomach, nourish your body and decrease your hunger.

• *Eat slowly.*

Take twice as long to eat a meal as you normally do. Chew more. Not only will you find smaller portions more tolerable, not only will you metabolize your food better— you'll feel more like a more elegant eater! And this is good.

One of my clients who started the program told me about having dinner with some friends at a fine restaurant, and being fascinated by an attractive woman sitting with an attractive man at a nearby table: "Sheila, this woman had would you would call a charming presentation of self. She smiled and talked with her companion in such a feminine way. And what struck me too was, she looked so lovely while she was eating. She'd put down her fork between mouthfuls, talk a bit, turn her attention back to her plate, have another bite. The way she ate was just sort of classy." Something to aim for!

• *Don't think in terms of "bad" foods and "good" foods.*

Bridget, a woman I worked with, said she's been on "probably two dozen diets" in her life, and each time, she followed some advice she's heard about snacking: "I work at home, so it's always easy, not to mention tempting, to run into the kitchen and grab something to nosh on. Every time I'm trying to lose weight, I do what they say and keep a plastic bag of cut up carrots and celery in the fridge so I can grab that when I'm starving or I want to put something in my mouth."

The problem? It doesn't work. "I hate eating raw carrots and celery! Just hate it! So I might do this for a day or two, and then the bag sits there until the vegetables get droopy and I toss it out."

She craves something satisfying, which is something sweet. When she was working the program and focusing on weight reduction, she adopted this better idea: "My husband and my son love ice cream and frozen yogurt, and we always have this in the house. And this took some training and determination and a lot of talking to myself, but I can get the satisfaction I need by just taking one spoonful of cherry vanilla ice cream or whatever. I get the sweet taste in my mouth, and it cuts the craving, and then I have no more."

Eliminating from your existence the "bad" foods you love is no fun. And it makes it more likely that you'll crumble and have a pig-out day eating a whole carton of the stuff. You can have a little of everything—as long as it's just a little.

• *Drink water.*

A lot of it. Yes, at least eight glasses a day, which amounts to about three of those medium-sized plastic containers of the bottled variety.

• *Move more.*

This is the calories-out part of weight loss. Exercising is great, of course. And we know that women (men too, for that matter) ideally should do some stretching to maintain or increase flexibility, some weight lifting to strengthen muscles and bones, and some aerobic activity to burn calories and promote heart and lung fitness.

However, if you have been near the coach-potato end of life for a long time, simply think right now in terms of *moving* more.

Many women I've worked with resist getting into fitness workouts, going to the gym, plodding along on the treadmill and so on. Or they start, don't stick with it long enough to get "bitten by the bug," and soon let all those worthy intentions fall by the wayside. I say, start smaller, think smaller. Just move more.

Some of the most encouraging reports concerning fitness tell us that a fair amount of calorie burning—and excellent overall health benefits—can be accomplished from doing the ordinary stuff of life, maybe with a little more oomph than you usually put into it. Like stretching while you're storing groceries or putting clothes away, taking the stairs instead of the elevator, putting on some music and dancing around a little while you're vacuuming. They also tell us that walking is a godsend for anyone who wants to stay healthy or who wants to lose weight or both.

All of the above, by the way—eating right, taking off the pounds, moving more—will do wonders for your cellulite, should you have any of that puckered, dimpled looking skin on your thighs or rear that you'd love to eliminate.

If your weight is okay but your shape is middle-agey

Katharine, in her early-fifties, was not unhappy with her weight, although she said it was a few pounds more than what she considered her ideal. Describing her body during the mirror test, however, she was depressed about it all: "The adjective I first thought of was squared-off. I have a sort of thick body these days. Soft in the arms and thighs. Then the second adjective I thought of was peary. Heavier-looking in the thighs and the rear than I used to be. Like everything sunk down."

She and her husband were in the process of divorcing. In talking about their joint possessions, Katharine wanted to keep the family photo albums, which contained many pictures taken in the years when their now young-adult children were growing up. Katharine told me: "I thought I'd be wistful and sentimental about the kids. I started looking through these albums again, for the first time in a long time, and what I was wistful and sentimental about and missed the most was my waistline. I actually had a waist back then!"

Katharine had that middle-agey body look.

Maybe you do too. Here's where some specific exercising might be of help, although you may not actually lose pounds and you won't change your basic shape. You also need to know that you can't decree where the weight is going to come off. Suppose you decide that losing seven or eight pounds should take care of the hippy problem or the big rear; then you lose the weight; and then maybe you discover that while your face and tummy are looking thinner, your hips and rear remain as pudgy as ever. What you *can* do is put effort into building up the muscles under the fatty areas. And to learn how to do that, search out a little help.

Not far from where I live is a neighborhood center that includes an exercise facility, with a room full of machines and weights and trained individuals who can offer some advice on how to use all that paraphernalia. The cost of becoming a member is a few hundred dollars a year, a lot less than many of the fancy gyms and workout spas that are all over. Maybe there's such a place near you. I'd urge you to put a little money where your mouth is, invest in a membership in one of these facilities, and get some advice and training that will get you started. There's an awful lot you can do at home, with inexpensive hand weights and the like, once you know what you're doing.

So what can help the middle-agey look? The women I work with typically complain about these areas:

• *floppy arms*

We women can actually get some great results from training—using free weights or one of those contraptions you'll find in a fitness center—that focuses on strengthening and toning the arms and shoulders. Wouldn't it be lovely to go sleeveless (or strapless) like you used to in the good old days?

• *the run-away waist*

Stick to your weight-reduction way of eating, keep up your aerobic type moving around, do some daily stretches, and you really can wittle down that waist. For us females, weight around the middle tends to come off faster than weight below the middle.

• *saddle-bag hips and thunder thighs*

Here's where aerobic exercise will help enormously. Can you get yourself to a pool on a regular basis and start doing (slowly at first) some lap swimming? Can you get religious about taking a two-mile, brisk walk on a daily basis, or slowly working up to one?

Suck it off

If all else fails—and I do mean you must give serious weight-loss eating and exercising a determined try—consider liposuction, the process by which fat is vacuumed from thighs, buttocks or other sections of the body. It works, but it costs a lot and it hurts a lot and you must find a very skilled practitioner.

If you cannot or do not want to lose weight, you are not alone! Under no circumstances should you become discouraged. In the following chapter, we'll talk a little about what your clothing can do for you in terms of dressing the shape you're living with.

CHAPTER 9

Your Clothes

Let us think for a moment about this matter of clothes, and what they do for you. Clothes can make a statement about who you are—an artistic type, a romantic type, an outdoorsy type, a vice president in a bank. They can cunningly show off what is fit and fabulous about your body, or just as cunningly disguise what is not so fit and fabulous. They can highlight the pretty color of your eyes or hair or skin, or perk up those features if they are not so naturally bright and gorgeous. Any or all of this is just fine.

Clothes should fit like a dream (this is a message I hope I have thoroughly drummed into you when we took a look in your closet). You should dress your body, at all times, in a way that makes you feel great and that gives you confidence.

I'd like you now to tuck another thought in the back of your head as you go about building up an excellent wardrobe: The clothes you wear should please the men you meet.

Most women dress to look good to other women. Invariably, a woman will buy a particular suit or dress because she knows another woman will tell her she looks great in it. After that, women dress to feel comfortable about themselves, or because they've been wearing certain kinds of clothes all their lives and they're set in their ways. Dressing for men is last on the list. Move it up! Remember the cause!

If for you the cause includes finding the love of your life, or holding on to him, you must pay heed to what it is that men like about the way a woman dresses. That does not mean throwing all your sense of personal preference to the wind, and pursuing some notion of "provocative." It *might* mean sometimes abandoning the safe-and-sure (aka, dowdy) and taking things up a notch, being a shade more adventurous and glamorous, looking like a woman who is interested in pleasing a man. This will be a challenge for you: Get yourself in another mindset, and start dressing for men, even if that notion burns you up.

So where to begin? We'll talk here a bit about camouflaging and highlighting and the basics, and about dressing for men.

"There are no designers who create for the forty- to seventy-year-old woman," said the feminist writer Germaine Greer, an annoyed-sounding sixty, in an interview. "We are still here, walking around, eating out, but we've got nothing to wear except, maybe a pink jogging suit." This is nothing new! The over-forty woman has been called The Forgotten Woman for years.

We all *hear* a lot these days about gorgeous "older women." We're supposed to be cheered by seeing "mature" celebrities like Cybill Shepherd and Sigourney Weaver featured in fashion layouts. And to be sure, those ladies are stunning and dress beautifully. But the real women I talk to are often disheartened and frustrated by the available clothes out there. Maybe the picture is not quite as dismal as nothing but pink jogging suits, but it's not encouraging either.

Said Margot, a woman I put through the program: "I actually used to like shopping for clothes. I played around with different looks, not all of them wildly successful, but I enjoyed the process. It hasn't been any fun in a long time. Everything I see in the department stores looks either very young and trendy or very boring." Some years back, well after her divorce and well into her career, Margot stopped playing and settled into her all-purpose wardrobe, pants suits and shirts.

I want to encourage you to recapture some of the pleasure, experimentation and fun you probably once enjoyed in making clothing choices. Most of us by this stage of the game have acquired a pretty solid sense of a handful of personal do's and don'ts. Maybe your shoulders are small and slightly sloping, and you figured out a long time ago that jackets and tops with some padding in the shoulders are flattering. Or stiff cotton fabrics add visual pounds to your heavy bosom, while silk blouses and sweaters drape more appealingly. By all means, stick to your shoulder pads and silks, but get a little creative.

If you've had to do major reimaging on your body, and that has involved finally getting serious about losing weight, you'll probably want to postpone a major wardrobe overhaul until you've got yourself looking the way you want to look. But I think if you have been religiously sticking to your eating and exercise plans, even if you're only halfway there you deserve a little reward, and a visible reminder of the big, big payoffs that the program will give you. Maybe it's time for a small splurge on something really pretty to wear—something sexier, more feminine, even more out-rageous than you've ever attempted before. Go for it!

Let's think now about reimaging your wardrobe. I mentioned earlier than when I'm helping one of my clients with her closet analysis, we try to keep and work with anything in there that's still remotely functional and has possibilities. Some of the sugges-tions that follow have to do with re-cycling old items for your own use, in ways you may not have thought of before.

DRESSING THE SHAPE YOU HAVE

Cast back over your notes from your last two mirror test sessions, when you took that good, objective look at your body and you came up with your "basic" shape. Your shape doesn't really change; there may be less *of* it than there once was, but the essential proportions remain. And there are ways your clothing choices—in particular, jackets, dresses and pants or slacks—will work well with or work against your overall image, depending on how thoughtfully you "dress your shape."

Here are some guaranteed-to-flatter styles for each. We'll eliminate the classic hourglass shape—average-or-taller height, average weight, evenly-proportioned with a defined waist, and shoulders and hips about the same width—and the tall and lanky, Katherine Hepburn shape. If it's your good fortune to be living in such a delightful body, dressing your shape isn't a big problem. Most clothes will look fine on you. If you are not one of those, you are probably:

• *bottom-heavy, or the pear shape*

Most of my clients, like many of us over-forty women, are dealing with the pear shape—larger on the bottom than the top, a little hippy, a little pudgy in the tummy, the thighs and the rear.

Jackets and dresses with small, softly rounded shoulder pads—not big, bulky and square ones—give you width across the shoulders, which is what you need. If you've got a good waistline, look for jackets with a bit of a nip at the waist and a bit of a flare at the bottom. These are so much more attractive on the curvy woman than boxy, straight-from-shoulder-to-hem tops.

Many bottom-heavy women believe the A-line skirt or dress is just the thing to make them look slimmer. In fact, the opposite is true: A-lines make you appear wider and shorter, so avoid them. Search out skirts that are tapered in at the bottom. Avoid pleated slacks (that you think you need to ease out over that tummy). A well-cut pair of flat-fronted pants (go a size larger, if you have to), with a side or back zipper, will make both your tummy and your behind look amazingly smaller and better toned.

A long vest, one that comes down over the rear, does great things for too-big hips or rear.

• *top-heavy*

If you are large in the shoulders, the unconstructed, loose-fitting, single-breasted jacket is a good bet for you. Get rid of the shoulder pads that seem to come with every other sweater or blouse these days; just snip them out. V-necks should look good on you. If your bosom is very large and droopy, stay away from prints, even in blouses and shirts.

To get a little width at the bottom, minimize a big bust, and present a more appealingly balanced shape, go for A-line or softly flared skirts.

And for really skinny hips or, as one woman put it, "the flat-as-a-pancake butt," pleated slacks are becoming.

• *short and round*

Here's a mistake I have discovered a fair number of women with this shape are guilty of: They don't realize that they are actually a bit shorter than they think they are. A lot of us lose a little height as we get older (and gain a little weight at the same time), but we don't make adjustments for that reality and we buy clothes in the "normal" departments when we should be trying on the "petites." Shop for your correct size, or be sure to have jackets and skirts adjusted by a tailor.

Look for jackets that aren't too bulky and boxy, and that reach your hips. Long skirts will not look well on you; knee-length or just above the knee is best. Slacks should be flat-fronted and well-fitted; stay away from pleats. Stay away from belts. Pair a jacket with a skirt (or slacks) in the same color.

- *petite*

You're overall small, slim and shortish. Tops and bottoms in different colors are not the best for you, if you hope to give the illusion of being a bit taller.

Long skirts and short (bolero or waist-length) jackets will cut you down in height, so keep your jackets fairly fitted and fairly long, around hip-bone length. If your legs are good, or even if they're not, keep your skirts on the short side, just at or above your knee.

- *big and solid*

If you're a large woman—tall, big-boned, but not over-weight—jackets that are long and narrow, paired with above-knee length skirts might look terrific. So will separates—a plaid jacket with solid-color pants or slacks.

- *big and full-figured*

In the last chapter, I said that many women have a great deal of difficulty losing weight. And some simply don't want to; they've spent a lot of years engaging in the battle of the bulge, and they're not doing that anymore, period. If you're one of them, fine. The good news is that you always can look smart, stylish and feminine, and that the clothes choices you make can do wonders for your reimaged self.

I actually think the full-figured woman has a lot going for her these days in terms of clothing options, at least in relation to what used to be available. The picture is far from grim! This is a part of the industry that is finally paying attention to the fact that we really don't wish to be wearing tents, and that dressing the heavy shape is not just all about comfort and covering up. At the same time, if you're overweight you can "work" your clothes to give the illusion of being slimmer, and that's going to make your image a whole lot more appealing and feminine. Here's what to remember, the simplest do's and don'ts:

Dark colors, solid colors and the same color top and bottom (in jacket and skirt or slacks, in stockings and shoes) look best. A loose, longish jacket (even mid-thigh length) with a shortish skirt may be terrific on you. Buy your correct size. Anything too tight—a jacket that you can't button, for example—will only add pounds to your image, and look anything but stylish.

Softer, lightweight fabrics are almost always going to be more flattering to your shape than thick, bulky fabrics. Rayons, gabardines, lightweight wools, even some knitted cottons can be worn in all seasons.

So those are some basics for dressing the shape you have. Now let's get more specific.

WHAT SHOULD BE IN YOUR CLOSET NOW

Remember the goal from your closet clean out? Everything hanging in there should fit you properly, look great on you, and be ready to pull out, put on, and go! And I said when we were analyzing your closet contents that even if you end up with only three outfits that meet that goal, it's okay. You'll build from there.

What you wear during the day has everything to do with the life you live. If you're working in a rather conservative field in a conservative office you'll have a basic wardrobe that's probably different from what the fulltime homemaker/mother is going to be wearing.

Let's assume for the sake of discussion, however, that at the end of your closet analysis you had nothing—zip—left in there that fit and looked great and that you could pull out, put on and go. And let's assume that your typical day includes leaving the house, doing things, meeting people—the ordinary stuff of life. At the minimum, and following the "dressing your shape" guidelines I've just outlined, I suggest you go looking for:

• one very nice, simple, plain jacket in a lightweight (if it's spring or summer) or mid-weight fabric, in a neutral color of your preference such as black, brown, navy or gray.

• one skirt and one pair of slacks in the same color and fabric as your jacket.

• two or three blouses, one silky and one white cotton.

• one very nice, simple, plain dress in your preferred neutral color and that you can wear with your jacket.

• one sporty/casual outdoor jacket (if it's fall or winter).

• one good coat (if it's winter).

As long as these items are well-made, fit properly, and look great on you, you'll have the bare bones of a number of sensational looks—many of which you will achieve by the smart use of accessories (more about this later).

DRESSING FOR MEN: THE DATING WARDROBE

Yes! We are going to think dating! If you're an unattached woman hoping to find a decent man—and I know so many of you are—prepare now for a social life that includes taking your fabulously reimaged self out for dates. Believe that they will happen, and get ready.

A woman I know, a cheerful, somewhat plump fifty-year-old who's been married for ten years to a man who never fails to look at her with the eyes of love, wears "going out" clothes almost entirely in the red family—rose, deep pink, fire engine. She's actually not especially crazy about these colors, but her husband loves her in red and believes she looks glowing and sexy. She said: "Oh, I think I'm just a pathetic old man-pleaser." I think she's smart.

You may be constitutionally incapable of wearing a color you detest just to please a man (that's fine too), but let us consider how you might bend a little further in that direction. As we noted above, if you're like most over-forty women, you don't dress for men; you dress for other women. If you haven't had a date in years, you *really* don't have anything like a man-pleasing wardrobe. Starting now, get yourself into another head set.

I could call this section "five easy pieces," because I think that's really all you need as the basis of an evening-out wardrobe. Here it is:

• *the perfect little black dress.*

Still a winner, still a classic. By the perfect little black dress I mean a dress in a beautiful fabric and a simple cut, a garment that can be dressed up or down. You will need one for summer and one for winter. If you don't have good arms, each of these should have a short or elbow-length sleeve; if you have toned up those arms beautifully, sleeveless is terrific.

I swear by my own perfect little black dress, and have for years. You will too, when you find one. You can tie the sleeves of a sweater over your shoulders, tie a great shawl around your shoulders, add a gorgeous jacket (maybe in a contrasting color), accessorize in a variety of exciting ways.

• *the perfect little jacket.*

Consider investing in a heavy silk or satin, lined, simply styled jacket that might be white or a soft beige or maybe red. Black, of course, is fine too. Pay particular attention to the length and the cut, according to your body shape.

• *the perfect day-to-evening suit.*

A simple, great-fitting suit—maybe in a soft crepe fabric, definitely not in a wooly fabric—can be glamorized up in all kinds of ways. If you are wedded to your pants suits, I urge you to purchase now a suit with a skirt. Men hate women in pants; men love women in skirts. Stick with a pants suit if you must, but first look for something with a skirt.

• *the perfect evening pants.*

I love swingy, loose-fitting, palazzo style pants in silk, crepe, rayon or maybe even a heavy chiffon. They are sexy-looking and flattering, they look like a skirt, they work beautifully with that silk jacket, and almost every woman can wear them well.

• *the perfect shoes.*

The perfect shoes for your dating wardrobe are high-heeled, the higher the better. Men *love* women in high heels. Sorry, but there it is. If the wrong haircut can make or break the beauty of your face, the wrong shoes can make or break the image of your outfit. Wear high heels, no matter how much the pain. This is where my clients almost always draw the line, talking about ruined feet and how no man's worth it. But I wear them down and get them in those heels. These shoes, and your stockings, should be the same shade as your dress, to produce a continuous flow of color and not detract from your leg.

Said clothing and shoe designer Michael Kors: "You could be fat or bloated or short and it doesn't matter, the shoe will still fit! With shoes there is no age." This is true, and another thing: You can transform almost any outfit by wearing a sexy shoe. Your legs look thinner, you look taller, you will walk in a more feminine manner.

Now comes the really fun part, the add-tos and dress-ups:

• *Wear a plain, white, scoop-necked T-shirt under your suit and look terrific.*

A woman I know bought herself an absolutely gorgeous pants suit in a dark and dusky charcoal, tried different blouses with it, thought the effect was a little more blah than it should be—and then went out and purchased a man's white, ribbed, U-neck undershirt, and was thrilled with the sexy effect this achieved. When you really get into reimaging, you start getting bold.

• *Buy a camisole.*

There are beautiful, feminine camisoles readily available these days, many of them lacy and delicate. Even if you're heavy and want to keep your arms under wraps, a camisole with your suit or pants and silk jacket can be dynamite.

Give some more thought to this matter of what to wear under your jacket. I was once helping a client dress for an evening out, and persuaded her to try the bra top of her bathing suit, which happened to be a shocking pink, with her very pretty but plain two-piece suit. She was in excellent shape with a nicely-toned midriff, and she looked sensational, and very sexy.

• *Hunt up a pretty shawl.*

I love large scarves or shawls, maybe with fringed bottoms, to wrap and tie loosely over your shoulders. If you have such an item, do, however, experiment with it before heading out for an evening. A lot of women, I have found, love the look of a large scarf but aren't comfortable wearing one. The draped evening scarf isn't going to do much for your dating image if you're always tugging at and rearranging it.

• *Think trendy.*

I'm not a big fan of trendiness when it comes to wardrobe basics—your clothes. With accessories, however, I think you can go a little trendy, look modern, have some fun and not break the bank. If leopard prints are "in," it doesn't cost much to pick up a small leopard print handbag or a belt, and spice up your basics that way.

• *Add a touch of color in the small pieces.*

A good wardrobe of basics in the neutral color you prefer—black, brown, navy, gray—is foolproof. Just the smallest bit of color—a small, red silk scarf tucked into a jacket pocket, maybe—gives it life.

• *Own a small evening bag.*

When it comes to handbags, do have a small and elegant purse for evening. It can be very plain, basic black leather, but nothing looks less appealing than going out for the night hauling around one of those big carry-alls or totes.

• *Jewelry is the finishing touch.*

You'll never go wrong with simple pearl studs in your ears, but—especially if yours is a big and solid or a heavy body shape—you can afford to get more dramatic. A long and rather large necklace, for example, looks terrific on a heavy-breasted woman in a simple black dress.

REIMAGING THE CLOTHES YOU HAVE

If at the end of the closet section of your self analysis you ended up with a number of items in that category we called "things I don't wear a lot but maybe can re-invent," let's consider now what you might do with them:

• If you sew or have determined to hunt up a decent tailor, re-fashion that dress with the frumpy sleeves into a sleeveless, maybe even a strapless. This isn't as hard as it sounds, and you might be amazed at the new life you'll give that outdated number.

• *Experiment with trims.*

Take that old suit or winter coat, buy a fake fur collar (some very excellent-looking ones are available these days, found in sewing or notion stores), and sew it on the lapels.

• *Indulge in a little button magic.*

Here's a quick-and-easy, down-and-dirty way to transform any outfit, and it's one of my favorite ways to update a blouse, a suit or a dress. Sometimes I just pin the buttons on for an evening to give the thing a new look. Try buttons that are a bit outrageous and fun, bright and glittery, even trendy. It's truly amazing how buttons can transform an outfit.

• *Re-hem a skirt.*

One of my clients had a longish skirt in a rather heavy fabric that she basically liked but never wore. We cut the skirt on an angle—one side shorter than the other—and re-hemmed it. It looks fantastic.

• *Pair the jacket of that dull, drab, tweedy but good suit you never wear anymore with a paisley, checked, flowered or otherwise outrageous skirt. I do this all the time, and it's a great look.*

• *Re-fit, re-fit, re-fit.*

I would be willing to bet money that you brought out of your closet one dress or suit that you really do like but can't or don't wear because it just doesn't hang properly on your body. Again, take it to a tailor and see if it can be re-fitted.

A GRAB-BAG OF RANDOM THOUGHTS

• If you've found one sensational style—the line of a dress, say, or a pair of slacks that does wonders—get more of it. Get one in an evening fabric or a summer print. Find somebody to make more of them for you.

Kay, one of my reimaging success stories, told me this: "Years ago, I used to sew. All dresses, nothing really hard like suits or coats. But I wanted to have a dress nobody else had, because you couldn't buy it. I found one Vogue pattern, a simple A-line, and I changed the neckline from a high round neck to a lower square neck. It was a fabulous look on me. And I made this dress probably twenty times, in all kinds of fabrics, some prints, some plain, sometimes with a three-quarter sleeve, sometimes short."

Kay felt she never looked better. These days, she's not into sewing anymore herself, but she discovered another great, simple style for her current shape, and found a seamstress in her neighborhood who'll make some copies for her at not much cost. A great idea.

When something really works, do more of it.

• Keep the boring-but-necessary items simple.

Don't clutter up your now nicely uncluttered lingerie drawer with lots of versions of those knee-length hose that are great for wearing under pants. Have a couple in the colors you need (black, gray, neutral or whatever), and don't bother with prints or different fabrics.

• If you have a "look" you like—outdoorsy, say, or Eastern—don't overdo it. Sometimes you can get the same effect with a piece of jewelry. Too much of a good thing is a bad idea.

• A rule of decorating says this: If, in a room, you have two blues that are clashing, add a third blue and like magic, all three will look lovely together. Sometimes this can work to gorgeous and dramatic effect with clothes, too.

A woman I worked with had a lovely turquoise top and a lovely peacock blue skirt that she never thought of wearing together. We found a kind of muted emerald long jacket, and all three pieces looked suddenly sensational.

• A turtleneck sweater in cashmere or a cashmere-like fabric is invariably dynamite on almost any woman.

• Have a plan when you head out to shop.

Think of the several items you've decided you should have, and look for them— specifically.

• Look good when you head out to shop for clothes.

Do you remember Beverly, the woman who described her closet-clearing a few chapters back? Among the items that she found depressing were purchases made on sale and those several outfits for fancy dress affairs that she never liked and paid too much for. Beverly said this, too: "Most of the time when I've gone shopping, which I don't really enjoy, I've been wearing my old jeans and my old sneakers or whatever. I think this actually had a negative effect. Looking and feeling the way I did, I kind of wanted to get out of there fast, and I made some rash decisions." Now she's taking the time to dress nicely, style her hair and apply attractive makeup before she hits the stores. A very wise idea.

• Put on your jewelry, and then eliminate some of it.

A woman I know, who usually dresses in elegantly tailored suits, wears tons of jewelry. She'll have on at any one time six or seven rings, several chains around her neck, a bracelet on each wrist, and rather large earrings. She pulls this off, somehow, without looking garish, and I think that's because of those elegant suits *and* because she has an outsized, bubbly, vivacious personality. Most of us, however, do not look our best laden down with all kinds of jewelry.

Jewelry is fun to wear, and it always fits. Less, however, is more.

• Have your one unique thing.

This isn't a suggestion for everybody, or a "must do." If you try too hard or belabor the idea, it won't come off. But listen to Rachel, one of my clients: "There's a woman I work with and I also often see in the evenings at various functions, some of them dressy affairs. I've known her for years. We've done a lot of socializing together. And she *always* wears around her neck a very thin, choker-length, little gold chain. This is whether she's in office clothes or a swim suit or an evening gown. Maybe she'll also have on a giant string of huge pearls or something, but always there's that little chain. It makes you wonder. Is there a history to it? Who gave it to her? Why does she never take it off? It somehow adds to her fascination."

Do you have your one unique thing, a signature piece?

• Avoid youthful fads.

Exposed lingerie straps might look modern and sexy on a twenty-two-year-old. On you they won't.

• If you possibly can, buy one really good thing from a good designer. Get the experience of wearing a piece of clothing that's well made, well cut, in a good fabric.

• Pay less attention to style and more attention to fit.

A woman who's very fond of blazer jackets realized that most of them didn't really fit her to a tee—in particular, the sleeves were always about an inch too long, something she thought she could just live with. I urged her to take those jackets out to the tailor and get them shortened. For a really polished, pulled-together look, your clothes must fit. Don't live with the too-long sleeves.

• Find the right length skirt for your body, and stay with it.

Experiment with the clothes you have or when you're trying things on in the store. Most women have one hemline that's right—just hitting the top of the knee, an inch or two below the knee, or wherever. Keep all your skirts right there; shorten one that's longer.

Are you feeling pretty good about your wardrobe? When you know that everything you have looks great on you, is stylish, and fits your body, nothing beats that, does it? And when you know that men are going to like the way you look, you're ready to go out there and find the one for you.

CHAPTER 10

The Presentation

Do you remember Rena, the woman I mentioned earlier, who wanted to turn herself into "a desirable woman?" After putting in a great deal of time and effort toward that goal, Rena looked quite lovely and appealing. Yet, two potential blind dates who spoke to her over the phone decided she wasn't the woman for them. Without ever laying eyes on her! They didn't like what they heard. From the friend who was trying to arrange the fix-ups, Rena learned that one of these gentlemen thought she sounded "too tough and scary" for him.

My friend Mary had a similar experience. She had spent the better part of one year on her reimaging program and had wrought small miracles in her appearance. Many pounds slimmer, with a flattering cut and color to her hair and some simple and pretty clothes, Mary looked and felt great. However, although her work and fund-raising activities gave her ready opportunities to socialize, Mary wasn't getting many dates. And she too had a friend who had decided to "find a guy for Mary." Nothing had proceeded past one meeting.

Both these women were neglecting aspects of their image that detracted from their appeal—from that charming presentation of self, as I like to call it. Rena, wisely, spent some time tape-recording her in-person and phone conversations, and admitted ruefully that she had "a kind of staccato delivery, I sound all-business." Mary was a ferocious gesticulator. Acting as her confidante, I pointed out to her that in casual company she looked as if she was on the attack—fingers jabbing, arms waving, brows furrowed.

Both women needed to learn some lessons in reimaging their presentation, and had to put into practice more feminine and appealing behaviors. Perhaps those are lessons that will benefit you as well. Think again briefly about that notion we discussed at the beginning of this book, the fifteen-second window of opportunity to make a good impression. You may look like a million bucks, but if you walk in a slumpy or masculine manner, if you talk in a way that men find "tough and scary," if through your body language you send out the vibe of a jittery, tense, angry or nervous female—you lose points, a lot of them!

I witnessed a dramatic demonstration of this truth just recently. One of the guests at a large cocktail party my husband and I hosted was a woman who had clearly put a great deal of thought and attention into her appearance. She wore an absolutely elegant midnight blue crepe suit, short skirt and longish jacket, and a shiny blue silk camisole top underneath. Small diamond stud earrings, which glittered beneath her very short, chic, swept back and beautifully highlighted hair. Excellent, understated makeup. I couldn't fault her looks—she even had on those sexy, high-heeled, strappy evening shoes that I do recommend (as you know). However, she walked into the room as if she were loaded for bear! She took big, long, loping strides; she looked around as if expecting to come face to face with her worst enemy; she appeared both threatening and as if she, somehow, felt threatened; she even kept her fists clenched. She looked scary to *me*! No men approached her.

She needed to learn a few ways to soften and enhance the great image she had going for her in many aspects. What those might be is the subject of this chapter.

The sound of your own voice

Do be aware of your voice. Most women don't realize how greatly a pleasing, soft, feminine voice can enhance their image, and what an impression it makes on a man.

If your tape-recorded talk revealed a less than appealing sound, do something about that. I am hardly suggesting that you adopt "a voice" that feels to you artificial, stagey or coy. But you *can* learn to modulate an off-putting, nervous- or anxious-sounding style. Here's how:

• Smile when you talk.

When you are speaking to someone over the phone, you'll sound better if you're smiling. This is true. Your phone partner, of course, won't see your face, but putting on a smile will make your voice sound happier and more inviting, thus making *you* seem more inviting.

• Lower your register.

Take the tone of your voice down a notch. Speaking in a somewhat lower, softer pitch is sexier. It also makes you sound more confident and pleasantly self-assured. And men like that. Men think they can tell a lot about a woman from how she sounds on the phone. Maybe they're right. My Henry said to me sometime after we had gotten to know each other that he knew he wanted to meet me from our first phone conversation. "You sounded so confident," he said, "I felt lucky having a chance to talk to you." What could be better than that?

• Speak slowly.

If you discovered during your analysis that you have one of those "staccato" deliveries, that you talk loud and fast and you're in a hurry to get it all out, work at slowing things down. Practice this with your tape recorder. You can read the newspaper or part of a book or a magazine article out loud, focusing on speaking slowly and clearly. Play your tape back, listen to yourself, and see if that sounds better.

- Don't use nasty words.

Do try to eliminate those "yep," "nope," and other clipped, getting-down-to-business shorthand comments that aren't terribly attractive.

Do try also to avoid lots of "Uh-huhs" and "Mmmms." Communication experts say that a little of this is to be expected, and gives a signal that we're really listening. If you have become aware, however, that nervousness makes you rush to fill in any silence with this "background noise," try to be a little quieter.

But *definitely* cut out unpleasant language from your repertoire. A woman I worked with had two favorite words she said all the time—"crap" and "bullshit." She'd often use these in a joking, amusing manner. But, I pointed out to her, they are angry-sounding words and unfeminine words. She did not sound appealing, attractive, or inviting when she inserted them in her conversation.

- Vary the inflection of your voice as you talk.

I mentioned earlier the woman who discovered she had a monotone speaking voice that made her sound tired or blasé. It will also make a woman sound bored, as if she's not particularly interested in knowing more about the person she's talking to. With a little practice, it's really quite easy to alter a monotone, all-one-pitch, conversational voice in order to sound more animated and thus more appealing. Radio and TV newscasters are trained to do this, and you may notice how one of those individuals vary the pitch of the words in the course of saying a sentence.

Of course, you do not wish to sound weird and as if your inflections have no connection with the meaning of your sentence. But talk into your tape recorder, practice getting a little more lilt to your delivery, and see if this doesn't improve the way you sound. Again, read something aloud and listen to your sound. Avoiding a monotone delivery makes you come across as a more interesting woman, a woman who has emotions, curiosity, and passion.

- Don't talk at the wrong times.

Do not interrupt another person when he's speaking. Do not cut into the end of his sentences in order to get out what you want to say. Listen!

The walk

Said Camryn Manheim, good-looking actress, size twenty-two, promoter of large-sized clothes for Lane Bryant: "When I got on television and people wanted to put me in beautiful clothes, I didn't even know how to wear them. There's a way you strut down the runway. There's a way you walk through your life that you have to learn."

I love that idea—the way you walk through your life—and I think she's right, you have to learn it.

- Practice the slow, sensual walk (once you get it, you'll love it).

Get a slight, ever-so-gentle swing in your hips. Practice the runway walk, the way those models do it—one foot directly in front of the other. At home, pretend you're on a runway and practice the glide, small steps with that gentle little swing.

Stand tall when you walk! Keep your back straight, your head up, and your shoulders back and down, not hunched up around your neck.

Walk into a room full of people that way, and pause for a moment as you look around with a smile. Do not scurry off into a far corner, seeking comfort and concealment. Give people a chance to notice you.

- Remember those posture tricks your mother taught you? She had the right idea!

I cannot recommend strongly enough that you put a book on

your head from time to time and walk around your living room balancing it up there. An old, tried-and-true lesson that really does wonders to remind you what it feels like to stand tall and straight, and to improve your overall posture.

Body language

Consider whether you'd be wise to reimage some body language basics. For example, do you need to learn these lessons?

• Don't speak with your hands.

Actually, some women can look quite charming doing this. They appear lively, expressive and fully engaged in their conversation; their "hand talk" somehow adds to their interest. Many women look simply nervous, however, or antsy and on edge. I hope you received from your confidante some helpful feedback about your own hand talk, and whether it was typically appealing or distracting. If you have concluded you tend to wave these appendages around too much, remember to tone things down.

Slow, graceful hand movements are feminine, sexy, inviting, and put other people at ease. Don't fidget with things, like your dinner napkin or your handbag. Be aware of where your hands are, and quiet them down. One woman on the program realized after watching a video tape of an evening's party in her home that her hands were always flying up to her face—she covered her mouth when she laughed, she drummed her fingers on her cheeks, she fussed at her hair. This was hand talk of which she had been completely unaware, and that she found most unattractive. She vowed to keep those hands still.

• Don't point your finger at your companion.

Men hate this gesture in a woman. It seems to them strident or accusatory. Maybe it reminds them of getting a scolding from their mothers. Make your conversational points without pointing that finger.

- Sit with your legs crossed gracefully.

Splayed open legs are nasty-looking on a seated woman. If your body work has left you with slimmer, trimmer thighs and calves, you're all set to drape one leg gracefully over the other.

- Sit up straight.

No slouching. No sliding down in your chair. Some of the most elegant women I know always sit forward in their chairs, their backs not touching the back of the seat. Clearly, they have excellent posture and strong lower back muscles to be able to pull this off. If you can't go that far, at the very least don't slouch or slump.

- Establish eye contact.

Give the person you're talking to your complete attention. But don't stare. I have noticed that some women—apparently having read somewhere this excellent advice about making eye contact—will focus their eyes on a companion with laser-like intensity, never breaking that connection. Too much of a good thing! The intense stare makes another feel not so much paid attention to as under the spotlight. It's uncomfortable. Good eye contact does allow you to blink sometimes, or look down at your dinner plate or whatever. (It does not allow you to be darting your eyes all over the room.)

Establishing good eye contact means you face the person you're talking to. In a social gathering, turn your body so that the two of you are face to face, not shoulder to shoulder. You'll present yourself as a more open and welcoming individual.

- Unfurrow your brow.

If you perpetually crinkle up your forehead while you talk or listen, or do that frowning thing that creates vertical furrows between your eyes, stop it. Again, you'll appear vaguely angry or annoyed, rather than intrigued and interested.

• Smile.

The best smile is the one that shows in your eyes as well as your lips, that looks as if you're smiling because you are happy to be where you are.

So now we've come to the end of the reimaging basics—what you need to do to get great-looking hair, face, skin, body, wardrobe, voice, walk and all the rest of it. The work is up to you. And you will do it! Now I want to put this one added thought into your head: You must *keep on* working at it, all the time, forever more.

The reimaging cause doesn't stop cold once you're feeling pleased as punch with how you look. You've got to keep it up, and that means caring for yourself, tending to yourself, maintaining the goal. And yes, you can say out loud once again: This is humiliating and annoying and insulting for an educated, accomplished woman! Doing all this fussing and focusing and obsessing about my image makes me feel like a jerk! I resent it!

Say that, and then get on with it.

PART IV
Changing Your Life: Dating and Beyond

Congratulations! You've done it!

You look in the mirror and feel sensational about the woman you see. You look fabulous. Maybe the best you have ever looked in your life. It's been hard, hard work, but you did it. You are loving the compliments that seem to be coming your way. You are enjoying the kind of respect and attention from friends, co-workers and men you haven't received in years. Feels great, doesn't it? Worth every bit of time and effort you put into the reimaging cause? You're ready to go into the world as an infinitely more confident and determined woman than you have been in a long, long while.

I'm not suggesting, of course, that over these past months, while you've been diligently working on the program, you have been holed up behind closed doors and now you will emerge into the daylight for the first time. Life went on; you had a job to go to, food to shop for, family to tend to. But I am guessing you have achieved now a new mindset, as well as a new look. It's a mindset that will let you meet and greet the world "out there" in a way you haven't in a very long time—as a world full of options and possibilities.

I considered calling this last section "The Big Payoff." What that payoff will be is up to you. Perhaps you remember the book published years ago, LIFE BEGINS AT FORTY. I can assure you from personal experience and the experiences of so many of my clients that life truly can begin at forty, fifty, sixty, even seventy. Yes, I've worked with several over-seventy women who determined there would be more to their days than playing bridge and talking about their aches and pains. One has started dating after her husband's death ten years ago, and is, she says, "having a ball!" Another decided to start a new business venture, and has done so with great success.

Are you ready? Of course you are. All that's necessary now is to decide what you want to do with your life. And if, for you, ideally that will include becoming involved with a good man, the remainder of this book may offer some ideas you should hear. We're going to talk about men—how to meet them, how to get to know them and let them get to know you, and how to encourage a relationship that leads to marriage.

If you're happily married or otherwise blissfully coupled, you need read no further. But I have felt compelled to write about "the man thing," for two reasons. First, as you know by now, it is so much a part of my own life story—from allowing myself to be demeaned, dominated and belittled by a father and a husband; from recognizing and then breaking the pattern to continue to seek out "the wrong man" and convince myself he was "the right man"; and finally, to gaining the self-esteem and confidence to attract and share my life with a truly wonderful person.

And my second reason: During the ten years between my divorce and my second, extremely happy marriage, as I developed my business as an image consultant, I became acutely aware of how difficult single life is today for women in their forties, fifties and beyond. I was shocked by the number of women who confided to me that they hadn't had sex in years, hadn't had an affectionate relationship in years, or were stuck in loveless, sterile or downright bad marriages. I was dismayed by the number of women who described lousy, awful, dreary dates; who said, "That's it! I don't like men, don't want 'em, don't need 'em! I'll live alone and get cats instead!" Said one: "I've dated a whole string of potential serial killers. No more!"

I met those women, and I continue to meet them, all the time.

And despite protests to the contrary, most of them *do* want something more. They want what I believe we all want, men and women both—a loving partner, for life, because that's the nicest and the healthiest way to live. Recently, an accomplished, intelligent, educated woman looked me up, saying: "Will you help me? I think at this point I'd even be happy with a stupid man in my life. Is it too late?"

It's never too late. And by no stretch of the imagination is "a stupid man" all that's out there for you. I'd be the last person on earth to say that we all need to *get* a man, *any* man, just to *have* a man. But achieving that solid, healthy, loving, lasting relationship may be the most difficult job you will ever have, a lot more difficult than the one you do now to make a living. Actually, I believe that finding the right mate is the hardest thing any of us ever does.

Here's a tale to give you pause: Vera Wang, the enormously successful designer of wedding gowns and other fantasy dresses, realized at one point some years ago that the demands of her business precluded a rewarding personal life. So she made the decision to remove herself from the day-to-day involvement in her company, and devoted one solid year to achieving that personal life. It was her goal, her new job. And she did it, finding a man she loved who loved her back, and marrying him.

Several women I have reimaged have followed the same path, actually taking time off from their job lives to focus on their social lives. I say, more power to them. And brava, Ms. Wang!

I am guessing that such dedication is not in the realm of possibility for you, for financial or other reasons. I hope you *will* take away from the examples of those women this message, however: Looking and feeling like a sensational woman will carry you a long way. But to reach the satisfying personal life you long for will take time, as well, and effort, determination and commitment to the cause.

In these final two chapters, I'll share with you some of the lessons I learned from my own experiences, and those of my clients. Most critical: Changing old notions and patterns having to do with your appeal to men may be the biggest hurdle you will face. But you can do it! And you can find what you want!

CHAPTER 11

First Forays: Beginning Your Reimaged Social Life

Bring on the men! But, you say, how?

You know, of course, that a man will not appear at your door, looking for you. So now, you will push your fabulously reimaged self out that door and go looking for him. You must be courageous, and more than that, assertive, even aggressive. This is no small task. You will not at all times feel powerfully self-confident, much less assertive or aggressive. Little demons of insecurity and fear of rejection will keep popping up, always ready to take over. Beat them back!

In this chapter I'm picturing the reimaged you, looking sensational, the best you have in years. You are ready for your first forays into a social life you haven't been in for a long time or perhaps ever, or felt was closed to you because you're not twenty-five anymore. You're wondering where to start, or how you'll handle these new challenges. I'd like to give you some suggestions about all that, beginning with the most critical power you should have in your arsenal: A good attitude!

Believe you will succeed. Attitude is half the battle.

Single life is hard at all ages; it's twice as hard after forty—but not for men! Some hard truths: The over-forty man is a real commodity. So is the over-fifty and over-sixty man. Usually, he's more successful, more confident, more interesting and more self-assured than a younger man. He's more egotistical, too. The unattached older man who likes women has more women than he knows what to do with. Again, he's not looking for you. You must look for him—and you will succeed, if you begin with the right attitude. Here's what I want you to do. Look in the mirror once a day and say:

"I look great. I feel great about myself. I will be successful. I will be courageous, determined, optimistic, strong, willing, and ready to explore all avenues in order to achieve my goals.

"I refuse to feel defeated.

"I will not give up until this job is done. I am going to change my life and I am going to find my partner. I am going to have a happy and fulfilled life. If I become discouraged, I will look in the mirror, apologize to myself, and get over it. I have made a decision to do this thing, and nothing will stop me."

Mentally put three or four exclamations points after those statements. Begin with the right attitude.

Ignore statistics

Perhaps you remember this alarming prediction popularized in the news a few years back: The unattached over-forty woman has a greater chance of dying in a plane crash than she does of getting married. To which I say: Hogwash! It is absolutely possible to find your man, whatever your age.

Decide you will stop yourself from excessive brooding over

dismal statistics relating to women—even, in the broader sense, *numbers* relating to women. Get beyond the thinking that goes: "I'm fifty-two. They say there are ten women for every one man. A fifty-five-year-old man doesn't want a fifty-two-year-old woman, he wants a thirty-five-year-old." The older man/younger woman thing happens, as we well know. Which doesn't mean that it will happen to you, or that a charming fifty-five-year-old won't long to be with your charming, feminine, appealing fifty-two-year-old self.

Ignore statistics and numbers!

LET PEOPLE KNOW YOU'RE INTERESTED IN MEETING AN AVAILABLE MAN

Nobody is going to arrange your happiness for you. But more than that, nobody is going to know you're looking for happiness if you don't tell them.

So many women think, "Well, my friends care for me, people see I'm unattached, they'll fix me up." This is not true. They may indeed care for you, but they are unlikely to *do* anything to further your social life unless you make your situation known. Especially if you present the picture (as so many of us do) of an accomplished, independent, taking-care-of-business-on-my-own woman, others will remain unaware of your wishes and needs. They'll assume you're doing just fine.

You must put out the word that you are available and interested in dating, and generally take a determined, clear-eyed approach to networking, or acquainting yourself with a group of people—men and women—who will take your interests to heart and whose interests you will take to heart. We must all help each other out here!

Dorothea, a sixty-five-year-old speech pathologist, widowed

for one year, had this to say: "I had a joyous marriage for almost four decades, I cared for my husband during his final illness, I mourned the loss of him—this man I grew up with, this man I had my kids with. Then I wanted a new love in my life. I was ready for that."

Nobody would say Dorothea could "pass" for thirty-five, or even fifty-five. Personally, she'd never consider having a face lift, she said: "It simply offends my sense of what you should do with your discretionary money, if you're fortunate enough to have any." Dorothea also looks marvelous, with an elegant, very personal style. In her work, she always wears beautifully structured suits in soft fabrics, such as very fine wools or crepes, along with crisply starched, white or blue-and-white striped dress shirts—not a look for everyone, but somehow perfect on her small-boned, well-toned frame. And then, since she has reimaged herself, she has acquired a small, quite glamorous bunch of evening clothes—dresses or two-piece designs in fabulous, muted colors and color combinations.

When she was "ready for a new love," she spoke to everyone she knew well and some she didn't know well, and mentioned her wish to meet a man: "I learned to be quite forthright, even blunt about this, and reminded myself there's nothing wrong with that. I'd say something like, 'Michael's been gone for some time now. We had wonderful years together. Now I'd like to meet someone new. Do you know anyone you think I'd enjoy getting to know and who would enjoy meeting me?' You can say that to people without in any way sounding desperate. I think I'm good company, I like being with people. And I know that I have, as they say, a lot to offer someone. So why not declare my availability?"

It paid off. A professional associate of hers introduced her to the man she's now married to, a widower, a sixty-seven-year-old cardiologist. (Who says older men don't go for older women?)

They spent their honeymoon in England, hiking in the Cotswolds.

So get the word out. Network. But understand that good networking begins with knowing whom not to count on, which—if you are divorced—may include your old social group.

ANALYZE YOUR FORMER SOCIAL SCENE, AND WHAT ABOUT IT STILL WORKS AND WHAT DOESN'T

If you are divorced, married friends from your pre-divorced life will tend to disown you. Many women (although not all, by any means) have had this experience: You no longer get invited to the couples parties. People you have known for twenty-five years don't call you. You hear on the grapevine that your ex and his new woman are socializing with the crowd that used to be yours. (And the more professionally successful your ex is, the more likely it is that he will receive the invitations and you will not.) Even if the man was a bum and everybody knew it, you still are not hearing from old married friends.

There are reasons for this. Some wives you saw socially may feel suddenly uncomfortable with you; you're a threat. Couples like to be around other couples, and so the unattached woman is persona non grata in that scene. Or, more compassionately, your old couple friends think *you* would be uncomfortable at the dinner parties or other festivities, and they believe it is kinder not to ask you. Perhaps they'll have you over for a dinner with just the two of them, which can leave you feeling like a very large third wheel, or to come by for a Thanksgiving meal with the family, which can leave you feeling like a stray, someone they feel sorry for.

Try not to brood about all this, to take it personally, or to become bitter and resentful. Decide who from your old life will probably remain in your new life—because you genuinely enjoy their company, they genuinely enjoy yours, and the connection is affectionate and strong. Let go of the rest of it.

This is a time of new beginnings.

FIND THE WILL TO ENTERTAIN

So many women coming out of a marriage or even divorced for some time have so many excuses about why a social life is last on their "to-do" lists. And it's often perfectly understandable—they're working fulltime, there are children to help with homework and put to bed, the car has to be taken to the garage. Life is exhausting! If this sounds like you, decide to re-think some of the excuses. Remind yourself that forging a new life will take effort and energy; put that effort near the top of your to-do list. You made time for your physical reimaging, because you embraced the cause. Now make time for part two, your social reimaging.

If people aren't inviting you places, or if you don't want to feel like the third wheel, get your own socializing going. Invite people to your home. Keep it simple, make it last-minute, pot-luck if that seems to make sense. Ask some co-workers over to watch football on a Sunday afternoon, send out for pizza or Chinese food. Make a paella or a pot of chili, invite some people you'd like to know better to come by and bring a bottle of wine.

The point is, when you have been part of a couple for a long time, and especially if he was the one who wanted out and you didn't, it's difficult to get used to *not* being part of a couple. You still think of the world as coming in pairs. Early after a separation or into a divorce—when, even though you're looking good these days, you may still be feeling socially shaky—the very thought of playing hostess on your own can be daunting. If you keep things simple and spontaneous, entertaining isn't such a trial.

You need to be around people in social situations. Make the effort to be a social creature, somebody others find fun to be with.

CONSIDER WHETHER YOU'RE UP FOR SOME ADVANCED NETWORKING

This is entertaining with the specific purpose of bringing together unattached women and unattached men. There's a little more of an agenda going on than is the case with the pot-luck-dinner kind of evening, but you can *still* have fun and enjoy yourself and not feel in any way desperate.

Let's assume you've got a pretty good, maybe even high-powered job. You live in a city or a large-sized community. When you stop to think about it, you really do know a lot of people, if only casually or as business acquaintances. And, if you have been working at expanding your social circle for a while and putting out the word, your Rolodex has been getting fatter (or your Palm Pilot has been getting fuller). Throw some singles parties—or if the sound of that makes you nervous, call them "new faces get-togethers."

Here's how it works: Gather together five or more single, attractive, trusted, "normal" women friends, and take turns hosting small cocktail or casual, buffet-style dinner parties in each others' apartments or homes. Decide jointly that you will commit yourselves to arranging one such party a month for one year, with each woman inviting two or three unattached men for a relaxed evening at one woman's apartment. Men love these invitations, and are usually quick to respond! Again, keep the food simple, but a bit elegant. Have the CD-player going.

I am a firm believer in the great possibilities such get-togethers hold. With not too big a crowd, circulating and talking and getting to know people is no strain. And, in fact, this is how I met my husband! He wasn't at the party, but a friend of his was, a new man with whom I had a wonderful conversation and who called me two days later suggesting I might enjoy meeting an old friend of his—who turned out to be my Henry.

DON'T SPEND ALL YOUR TIME WITH OTHER WOMEN

Girlfriends are great, for comfort, support, letting down your hair. And women compatriots in the dating and mating games of life, your networking and get-togethers pals, can be tremendously useful. But don't slip into a social life that revolves exclusively around your female friends.

Martha, a reimaged forty-five-year-old never-married college professor, enjoyed her many close friendships. As she considered ways to reimage her social life to go along with her tremendously attractive new appearance, she realized that for years she had been spending all her after-work time with family members and friends. These were good times, to be sure—vacations in Europe with her three closest friends (also professors, also unattached women), holidays and weekends at her sisters' homes.

They were women-only times. And they were, Martha also realized, just a little too comfortable, a little too predictable. Perhaps, she thought, they were also something of a copout, a way of telling herself, "I'm busy, I have things to do, I have a social life." Martha determined to make some changes.

My message is: Enjoy your female friends, but don't make them your only social outlet.

AT AN EVENING EVENT, DON'T CLING TO OTHER WOMEN

This is part two of the above suggestion.

A number of the women I have helped through their reimaging programs have active evening lives. Some are professional women, some are involved in civic affairs and committees. They receive invitations to events which would be wise for them to attend, or which they can't avoid attending. Many of them find it uncomfortable to go as a solo act. They want the company of another woman, someone to sit with.

My advice is, first, go! If you receive an invitation that you think you can safely turn down (nobody will miss you, there will be no professional consequences if you're not there), accept it anyway. You never know whom you might meet. And second, go with a woman friend if your nerves really can't stand the thought of walking into a black-tie or other fancy affair on your own—but peel off from each other as soon as you can.

Sitting alone is good. You will be compelled, perhaps out of sheer discomfort, to start talking to strangers, who might turn out to be a lovely couple who become your friends and who know a great guy you might like. Alone is good because men do not like to confront women in packs, or even in pairs. (In this regard, not much has changed from your high school days.)

ACCEPT THE FACT THAT YOU MAY HAVE TO MAKE THE FIRST MOVES

I said at the beginning of this chapter that the reimaged woman has to learn to be assertive, even a touch aggressive. She does. Many of us have read all the "rules" on how to snag a man; we can hardly have escaped hearing about, at least, the enormously popular advice put forth in recent years that advised a woman to be hard to get—never accept a date for Saturday later than Wednesday, don't return his calls, let him call back, and so on and so on. Maybe that approach works for some, but I'm quite sure it does not work for the over-forty woman. It really doesn't. (In the next chapter, I have more to say about this matter of rules! Because there are some we need to remember.)

Make the first moves. Most of us have trouble being aggressive, putting ourselves forward when it comes to men. We've been raised to be "nice girls," "good girls." Here's another sad truth, however: In a social situation, such as a large party or a roomful of people, if you stand back and wait for a man to approach you, most likely you will remain there, standing alone. Again, call it unfair, declare it everything that's wrong with the world today, but most unattached men will approach the unattached younger women at any gathering. No getting around it, we *do* live in a youth-obsessed culture. The younger woman may have the luxury of waiting for that attractive man to come sailing her way. You do not.

Am I flying now in the face of all my previous encouraging words about ignoring numbers, forgetting statistics? Not really. The fifty-year-old gentleman may be entranced by your fifty-year-old self, once he's really taken a good look at you. In fact, he may become absolutely smitten with you. But nature being what it is— or at least, men being what they are—his eyes are likely to land first on the thirty-five-year-old in your way. So accept that *you* may have to put *your* best foot forward, first and fast.

Let me give you an illustration of what I'm talking about. It's a rather extreme example, of a rather particular kind of woman, but it's a telling one, with some lessons you need to learn. My husband and I hosted a large cocktail party, part of a fund-raising effort related to a political cause to which we were committed. Making my phone calls to extend the invitations, I was bemused—and utterly fascinated—to note that two of the women on my invite list questioned me intensely about this coming affair. Who would be there? they wanted to know—specifically, how many men, what men, single or married? Before they even accepted the invitation, they were "casing" the situation, deciding if it would be worth their while to attend. What was going to be in it for them?

They did come to the party, and I watched these two women in action—walking up to the available men, engaging them in conversation, "playing politics" to meet a man. They went about their socializing like a job. And they had a wonderful time! The men loved them! Some other women stood on the sidelines and waited for men to come up to them...and waited and waited.

Watching these two women go to work, the term vultures came to mind (to my mind, that is, but not, from all appearances, to the mind of any of those charmed men who were "hit on"). And yet, and yet...those women clearly came to the party with the goal of meeting an unattached, powerful, successful, and wealthy man, and they accomplished that goal. What happened later? Who knows? Men are flattered by a woman's interest in *their* interests, but pretense doesn't hold up to the test of time. Feigned interest is apparent sooner or later, and anything but attractive. Still, there's no possibility of "what happens next" if the man whose attention you hope to attract can't see you across a crowded room.

Make the first moves.

WORK THE ROOM. LEARN TO FLIRT.

Again, let's assume you find yourself at a large gathering, and you're in the company of many people you don't know. Work the room. Flirt.

Flirting has a bad name. It conjures up images that suggest coyness, or doing tricky little things with fluttering eyelashes, or other actions and attitudes we find phony and unpleasant. But what I mean by flirting is really just being approachable; it's anything *but* projecting a seductive come-on.

Being approachable starts with having a warm, friendly look on your face. Walk into a room with your head up, make eye contact with people, smile. Be careful not to project that look I did, as a friend pointed out to me—the look that says, "Come near me and I'll kill you!" How well I know what a difficult lesson that is to learn!

Out of shyness, and enormous insecurity, I appeared to be a snob. My nose was up in the air. So often even the newly reimaged woman will enter a room full of strangers looking aloof, distant, unapproachable, gazing up at the ceiling or down at the floor or out the window. Not smiling. Giving off the impression that she'd rather be anywhere else but where she is. It's all purely defensive, an effort to protect herself from being rejected.

Be aware of that impression. And remind yourself that each and every one of us gets rejected sooner or later. Such is life. But do not *set yourself up* for rejection by appearing intimidating and unapproachable. You may be tied up in knots inside, you may be fearing the brush-off, you may even be wishing you were anywhere else but where you are. Nevertheless, walk in and smile. Walk up to a man and start a conversation. Remember the lessons you learned when you were considering your presentation. That's working the room, doing a little flirting.

Here's another thought to keep in mind that will help: Many men are insecure too. We women don't always appreciate that reality. A woman thinks, "Well, he's not coming over to me, clearly he's not attracted." This notion was actually put forth in one of those wildly popular and widely read "how to get a man" books published in recent years. If he's not approaching you, said the authors, don't tell yourself he's just shy; the fact is, he's not interested. Wrong, I say! A lot of men really *are* rather shy and lacking in social confidence. They don't know how to deal with us. Get the right attitude. Assume the positive: The attractive man you would like to meet really would like to meet you.

HAVE SOMETHING TO SAY. USE CUE CARDS IF YOU THINK YOU'LL GO BLANK.

Having made your move, it's all too easy then to feel tongue-tied. What to say?

Have some conversation-opening lines, fail-safe questions, or ice-breakers ready to go. Write these on an index card, if that will help, glance at them and refresh your memory before you enter a roomful of unfamiliar people. What your ice-breakers should be will depend on the situation. Obviously, you'll want something better than "Do you come here often?" But you might have ready an amusing, brief anecdote about how you met your host and hostess, or whatever—some comments that are appropriate to the occasion and that will get the talk started.

And then: This may sound insulting, it may sound obvious, but be well read. Read or at least scan the daily newspapers, including the business and sports sections. Be informed about current events. Men really respond quite positively to women who enjoy discussing—and have something to say about—what's going on in the world.

HAVE SOMETHING ABOUT YOU THAT MAKES YOU DISTINCTIVE, UNIQUE.

Now, this is a sweeping bit of advice, so sweeping that it almost defies getting down to specific suggestions. But let me tell you something I heard from Claire, one of my clients, a woman in her late-forties, divorced for many years, the mother of a teen-aged son. Claire had been feeling like Invisible Woman for some time, even to her son! He loved her, of course, and he was aware that she was a bank vice president, but he didn't seem to take her very seriously, didn't seem to *see* her as an interesting person in her own right.

Out of the blue one day, Claire suddenly said to her son, "Did you know that I can stand on my head, without my feet touching the wall?" She proceeded to do this. Far from being mortified at the sight of his mother upside down, the boy thought it was pretty neat. After that, he sometimes asked her to demonstrate this feat to one of his friends. Claire thought she had underlined the fact that she was a *person*—an interesting, perhaps even slightly eccentric person—not just a parent, and had garnered a bit more respect and attention. She thought that lesson had something to tell her about the reimaged social life she was trying to achieve, and about attracting a man.

No, she didn't start standing on her head at dinner parties. She *did* start to think about Unique Claire—what she had, what she knew, what interested her. An impassioned armchair archaeologist all her life, she found interesting ways to introduce this enthusiasm into conversations. Men do like to talk about themselves! But they also like to hear women share their own genuine interests and talk about "real things" (not kids, ex-husbands, or relationships). Another aspect of Unique Claire: She had a small collection of antique, rather large, quite beautiful cameo pins, and she decided to show them off, sometimes accessorizing an elegant dress only with gold stud earrings and one of her cameos. They were attention-getters.

The point: Try to display something about you that's a little different from other women, a statement about yourself. It may be ever so little or slight—but "a something" that sets you apart from the crowd, "a something" that makes a man think, "That's an interesting woman."

TAKE A CALCULATED RISK. TELL A MAN WHERE HE CAN REACH YOU.

When I began my first job, I was given a business card to distribute. It looked "all business." Later, when I finally started to do more socializing, I had another card printed—this one, a small, elegant and feminine card, blue script on a cream background, just my name and address and number. Definitely not an "all business" card. I found it quite comfortable to hand my card to an individual I'd just met, saying simply, "I'd love to talk to you further." A calculated risk, yes, but my new acquaintance could say he'd also enjoy talking to me again, or he could simply accept the card and smile and make no commitment whatsoever—and no one came away embarrassed.

Consider whether you might want to adopt this tactic, all part of packaging yourself.

A FEW HARMLESS TRICKS NEVER HURT.

Without shame, I applaud any and all gambits, however well-worn, that will cause a man to stop, look and listen.

My friend Phyllis told me this story. Having completed the program, looking wonderful and feeling confident, Phyllis was doing her power-walk around the Central Park Reservoir in New York City early one morning when she passed an attractive man jogging in the opposite direction. They exchanged glances; he kept on jogging. Phyllis stopped, thought a moment, then turned around and trotted after the man. Catching up to him, she put her hand on his arm and said, "Charles! How are you?...Oh, I'm so sorry, you look exactly like an old friend of mine." The attractive man apologized for not being Charles. They had a little conversation then about the best times for jogging and about the relative benefits of jogging versus power-walking. Phyllis said, "Well, maybe I'll see you here tomorrow." The attractive man said, "I'll look for you."

Phyllis played her little harmless trick. Why not? More power to her!

Pretend the man you'd like to meet is someone you think you know.

On the jogging track around the reservoir, pretend to be a bit injured, slow down and hobble a bit, looking like you could use his helpful hand. (Phyllis announced she didn't have it in her to go *that* far!)

In the men's department of a store, ask him to let you hold up a tie next to his jacket to see how it looks, or ask what size shirt he takes, because he's about as tall as your brother.

Later, when you are dating, there will be no tricks.

LEAVE YOUR HOME! GO OUT!

So, I have been talking about parties, large social gatherings, working the room, and maybe you have been saying to yourself: "*What* parties? *What* social gatherings? *What* rooms?!"

Perhaps such doings are not part of your life, or your lifestyle. Or, perhaps with your new focus on socializing you have been meeting some charming new people, even making some good new friends. Since you have been putting out the word that you're interested in dating, you have had several introductions to eligible men. But an available man who appeals to you has not been among them. So now I say: Men are everywhere! They really are! Everywhere, that is, except sitting in your kitchen, looking for you. So leave your home.

Go out!

Go!

First, a word about personals ads: Placing an ad in the singles column of your local city magazine might be worth a try. My friend Betsy ran two ads, requesting a brief bio and a picture, and received over one hundred responses, to her great surprise. She eliminated all but fifteen, for a variety of reasons; spoke to those fifteen over the phone, met five in person, and has been dating a lovely man for two years. Betsy, who is fifty-three and looks absolutely marvelous, fudged on her age and described herself in the ad as forty-six. She reasoned that a man in his fifties might automatically skip right over one that listed her true age. The lovely man she's seeing is fifty-one, thinks the world of her, and admitted that he might not have pursued her ad if he had known she was fifty-three (as he does know now).

Lying about your age is not something I recommend (more about this later), but in this situation it might make sense. If you go the personals route, do be careful about the responses you receive, try to check them out as thoroughly as you can, and always meet in a public place, such as a restaurant.

The following, how-to-meet-men suggestions you really know already. But we will list them here for a couple of reasons. First, you must think about how to meet men, and where they might be, in a conscious, planned, pro-active manner. And that is probably something you haven't done in a long while, and probably something that strikes you now as terribly artificial.

This is what Annmarie, a forty-four-year-old self-confessed "workaholic" career woman, told me: "When I was in my early twenties, recently out of college, just starting my first job, living in my little studio apartment, no boyfriends in sight, I figured out how I might meet guys. I joined the Sierra Club, joined a church, joined a choral society. I volunteered in a program working with troubled teens, because a friend of mine did that and met a very nice fellow there. I did all kinds of things, most of which I did for the sole purpose of finding a guy!"

She did meet many of them, married one, divorced him some years later, and soon found herself absorbed with her climb up the corporate ladder. Now—looking quite gorgeous after the program, feeling quite good about herself, determining to develop a social life that, ideally, involved love and romance—she was embarrassed to be focusing on the old, how-to-meet-a-guy thing. "It's so juvenile," Annmarie said, "it feels like scheming and plotting. It feels like a step backward. And I hate the idea of doing something only because I'm trying to meet a man! It's pathetic!"

I gave Annmarie a stern talking-to. That's the kind of thinking she needed to beat back, and you do too. Call it juvenile, if that reassures you that you really are an adult woman who knows better. Consider it scheming and plotting, if you want. It is, however, not pathetic. It is not a step backward. It is a step *forward*, what you must do to increase your options and chances of finding the man you want. It is good to say all this out loud!

There's another reason I want to offer you the suggestions that follow. As you will see, several of them call for laying out some money and setting aside some time, and for those reasons they may not come naturally to mind, or you'll be inclined to dismiss them. But think about this: You were willing to spend time and money on the program, on your physical reimaging. You accepted the fact that such an outlay was necessary for the greatest results. Accept now the fact that spending as much time as you can possibly carve out of your busy life, and spending as much money as you can possibly afford, almost certainly will be to the good. Consider it another chapter in your investment strategy. Sure, you might bump into a wonderful fellow while taking the bus to work one morning, but stack up better odds in your favor.

And let us call a spade a spade, and say out loud that placing yourself in some "up-market" situations increases the likelihood you'll meet an "up-market" man—a successful, accomplished and financially comfortable man. If the right man for you isn't necessarily going to be wealthy or what the world considers successful, if you're not even thinking along those lines—wealthy and successful isn't so bad either!

So let me now flat-footedly, unapologetically give you this run-down (call it embarrassing, call it obvious, call it scheming) of a few good ways to meet men:

Go to political parties and campaign committee meetings. Ask how you can get involved helping candidates.

Go to church. Hunt out a religious group or affiliation that appeals to you *and* that hosts singles parties or groups. If you're not looking for God, consider that some men you might meet in such a venue aren't looking for God either; they're looking for a nice woman.

Go to tennis courts and golf courses. If you don't play, take some lessons. Tennis, for some reason, seems to attract terrific men. Go to a driving range where you can hit buckets of golf balls, and maybe ask for some advice from a man in the next lane. Take one of your vacation weeks at a tennis or golf clinic, improving your game and meeting fellow enthusiasts.

Go skiing, but avoid the ritzy resorts—they're populated by very gorgeous, very young women who define the term ski bunnies.

Go to sports events. Pick a sport—basketball, football, baseball; get into it, learn about the team and the players, maybe invest in season tickets. Men like women who like sports.

Go to a spa, such as Canyon Ranch in Arizona or the Berkshires, for exercise, relaxation and socializing. *Very* pricey, but they do offer specials. And interesting men actually do go to these places.

Go to a Club Med. Ask a travel agent about the most popular ones that cater to an over-thirty-five singles crowd.

Go out and join a specialized singles group, such as a chapter of the Single Gourmet, where people get together to cook and eat. You may meet mostly women, but you're expanding your networking possibilities.

Go on an outdoor adventure vacation—river rafting, mountain trekking, sky diving and the like will put you in the company of adventurous people, including some dashing men.

Go to Las Vegas. Take a friend, look for a good plane/hotel

package, and enjoy this amazing place. Many single men love Las Vegas, not to gamble but just for a weekend getaway and some golf.

Go to wine tastings.

Go to Divorce Anonymous meetings or Parents Without Partners meetings. (You *do* need to be a parent for this second one—that's not something you can fake!)

Go to the opera or the symphony, and visit the bar area between acts and buy yourself a glass of champagne. Many men go alone to concerts. Many men love the opera.

Go to museums, by yourself. Become a member of your favorite museum, and attend the special events often offered to members.

Go to art galleries on the weekends. Put your name on their mailing lists and get invited to their openings. Go to those.

Go to financial seminars, advanced ones, offered by brokerage houses. Ask informed questions.

Go to bookstores, browse. Sit in their coffee areas if they have them, have a cappuccino, read with one eye and keep the other looking out for men. Ask a man what he's reading.

Go to steak restaurants where business types lunch. Go with one friend, smile, look approachable.

Go to a gym, early in the morning or at night. Look clean and wholesome. Full makeup and "sexy" workout clothes with thongs look obvious and trashy. Ask a man for some help with a piece of equipment.

You get the idea. Put yourself in places where men will be, and then put into practice the attitudes and actions—be brave and bold! flirt! take a calculated risk! play a little harmless trick!—that will help you change your life.

One more thought, which might sound like the opposite of doing something/going somewhere for the sole purpose of meeting men:

Go out and do something you really enjoy. Or, go out and do something you have always wanted to try. Give some thought to this idea. Were you an impassioned, serious amateur water color painter in your younger days? Have you let that enthusiasm go by the boards, because "real life" matters have taken precedence over the years? Decide you will carve out some time to resurrect your old hobby, but don't indulge in it only in the privacy of your home. Sign up for a painting class. Browse around art supply stores—looking great, of course.

Have you always loved flowers and promised yourself that someday you'd get serious about trying to grow them indoors? Make the time to get serious about it now. Buy some potted plants, start to inform yourself, and then go out and join the American Gloxinia and Gesneriad Society or the orchid-growers association you read about.

Do you love singing in the shower and in the kitchen, and know you sound pretty good? Is there a choral group you can join?

Do a thing you enjoy or always wanted to try, put yourself in the company of other people who enjoy the same, and it stands to reason that you'll increase the odds of meeting a man who shares your enthusiasms or your values. Here's an example:

Barbara, one of my clients, had worked hard on her reimaging program. After one year, she was, as she described it, "looking sleeker and slimmer and more polished. Standing taller. Feeling calmer and more confident. For the first time in my adult life I had the wardrobe I really wanted—simple, classic stuff, not a whole lot." And then she did something she'd always wanted to, and something she had never felt quite ready for before:

"I've always been interested in meditation, by the idea of being a prayerful person, so to speak. And I always wanted to go on a long retreat to a 'quiet house,' or a monastery. Someplace in a beautiful setting with hiking trails, where I could spend the day in this peaceful, healthful way and go to morning and evening services."

For her vacation that year, she went on her retreat. And there she met the man she married twelve months later.

If you have read through this chapter, and you are musing on the suggestions and bits of advice, and your first forays into a fuller social life are still to come, I'd like to offer this added thought: Everything I've been talking about will come easier and more naturally and feel more comfortable than it reads on paper.

Something quite wonderful happens when you've applied yourself diligently to your reimaging, something of an almost spiritual nature. I've observed it again and again among the women I've worked with, and I felt it in my own life. The world begins to seem like a sweeter, more welcoming, more knowable place. You see the positive in other people, just as you've uncovered the positive in yourself.

You appreciate the struggles we all face, each in our own way, and you feel greater tolerance and compassion for this thing called the human condition. It's a kind of awakening. See if you don't experience it.

CHAPTER 12

Relationship Realities for the Over-40 Woman

You have met an attractive man, or maybe more than one. From the early signs, you think there is the possibility of something more than a date or two—the possibility of romance.

Or, a mutual friend or one of your new acquaintances from your get-together parties has given your name to someone, and this someone calls and suggests an evening out.

How do you handle yourself?

How do you read signs and signals correctly?

How do you encourage a relationship you wish to develop?

I thought of calling this chapter "Sheila's Rules of Romance for the Over-Forty Woman." But "the rules," as we've come to hear about them, seem to be largely about playing certain games—tricking a man into marriage, even sometimes by acting in ways that go against your own decent instincts. They're about making your moves, in a highly calculated manner, until the poor dumb fellow just can't stop himself from falling madly in love with you. While I am all in favor of a woman's consciously determining to meet and attract a good man—and making her moves!—I also believe that tricks are a bad idea. They don't become you. And they don't work in the world of women and men who have had some adult experience of life.

So consider the following thoughts not a set of rules to follow—do A, B, C, D and bingo, love and marriage are yours.

Think of them as some suggestions that are appropriate to your time and place in life (and to your reimaged self), and that take into consideration some of the uncertainties that often bedevil the older unattached woman.

If you have not been dating for many years, or if you were previously emotionally bruised and battered in a marriage or a relationship, you may experience a mixed bag of feelings now that do anything *but* bolster your confidence. Before you get to know a new man, it's normal to be gun-shy, even apprehensive or suspicious. Normal, too, to feel insecure all over again (the old demon to keep beating back), to wonder what to say or how to conduct yourself.

You're unsure of the signals you are receiving: Does this man like me? Is he "coming on to me?" Is he just being polite?

Sad to admit, but you may feel initially as nervous as a teenager out with a boy for the first time.

All this will get better over time.

Remember these thoughts:

RECOGNIZE THE MAN YOU SHOULD (PROBABLY) AVOID IN THE FUTURE.

If he reveals in the course of your first evening together or early on in your relationship that he hated his mother, forget him. Run, don't walk, in the opposite direction. A man who maintains a powerful aversion toward the first woman in his life usually ends up with powerful problems about all women.

If he flirts openly with other women in the street or in the restaurant, forget it. Don't see him again.

If he talks about his monster of an ex-wife on the first date and about the divorce that sucked him dry, move on.

If he's heterosexual, over-fifty, and never married, accept the fact that this is a man who has an aversion to making a commitment to women and will probably never want to marry you either, and decide if you can live with that.

If he's recently separated, be certain that you think *very* highly of him and his good qualities before you agree to continue seeing him. Accept that you will probably have to sit through his long, rigorous divorce, a process that might take a couple of years. Understand that he may not be a good bet, if you are interested in marriage.

Some no-longer-married men can't wait to hook up with a new wife, anyone. This is the man who can't stand being single, and who is probably much too needy and dependent to make a good partner. Many other newly separated men, mainly those who have come out of an unhappy marriage, are eager to date as many women as possible for the first year or two, and to enjoy an extended period of "having a fling," to "get out there and live a little." They also like to test their manly appeal by approaching much younger women. A separated or divorced man with any real substance, however, rarely wants to marry one of those younger women. He comes to realize they have little in common; also, it's highly unlikely he wants to start a family all over again.

The point is: You have a goal in mind, and you must not let yourself be distracted from it. Don't squander your valuable time on any man who is bad news, or on one who clearly is not going to be emotionally available until way into the future.

DON'T PLAY COY AND HARD TO GET.

If a man calls for a date and you know he is some one you would like to meet or get to know better, accept the invitation. If the invitation is for dinner that evening, four hours hence, accept. Don't play any games or listen to any voices in your head that say he should have called five days ago, or you shouldn't seem overly eager, or if you're so available it will look as if you don't have a life.

The only question on your mind should be, "Am I free?" If you are, say, "Dinner sounds lovely. I'll see you at seven."

IF YOUR FIRST IMPRESSIONS ARE LESS THAN POSITIVE, DON'T BE OVERLY CRITICAL.

Your friend-of-a-friend, the man you've heard wonderful things about, shows up looking less than gorgeous. Maybe he's short, a little potsy. Maybe he seems not terribly sophisticated, even a bit nerdy. Of course you will not register on your face any disappointment you're feeling. But make an even bigger effort—to be courteous, accepting, willing to be pleasantly disabused of your first impressions. One hour into your evening, or one date later, you may realize you are fortunate enough to be in the company of a kind, intelligent, witty human being.

"Well," you're thinking, "of course I'm not going to be rude or dismissive. I'm an adult. I know that character counts and surface appearances are deceptive." I want to offer this bit of advice about first impressions, however, because I've learned from working with many of my clients that a woman will sometimes mentally give a new man the brush-off from the get-go! We become fussier as we get older. We're choosy. We make up our wish-lists of the perfect man. And he doesn't exist.

But a woman will also write off a new man as a possibility, I believe, out of defensiveness, self-protectiveness, fear—an instinct to climb back into her solitary cave, because at least there she knows the score.

Listen to Moira, a woman who found herself doing just that, and then had the good sense and insight to realize her true motivations: "Bert, whom I'd never met before, came to pick me up. He had suggested dinner and then the theater, which was actually a pretty nice first date. And as soon as I opened the door, I decided he wasn't my type. Like I had a *type*! Me, who hadn't been out on dates in years! And the evening was perfectly pleasant, but I was emotionally closed off, I guess you'd say. And I didn't hear from him again after that, to my regret.

"It was a way of keeping myself safe, I realize that now. If I told myself right off the bat that this man wasn't for me—well, clearly he'd never get the chance to decide I wasn't for him, would he?"

If you have no reason to suspect the man you've just met is truly bad news (see the above, on men to avoid like the plague), he warrants the benefit of your doubt, and maybe a second and a third chance. He may turn out not to be a man for you in the long run, but will become a caring friend. Or, you may realize a female friend of yours might be a perfect match for him. (Remember, we all have to help each other out here!)

There's also this: Men don't change deep down. You will never turn a domineering, controlling man into a better one. Surfaces, however, can always be modified and improved, and a good man with whom you enter into a more long-term relationship might be perfectly amenable to some reimaging suggestions.

On our first date, my Henry showed up wearing sneakers and a sweater with a large hole. Clothes are not terribly important to him. He dresses quite nicely these days, in part thanks to my help.

ENJOY YOUR DINNER.

Dining out with a man, especially early in your (potential) relationship, should not be a time for worrying about your diet—or obsessing about yourself in any way, for that matter. When you were working the program, self-absorption was a good thing, necessary to keep you motivated and believing in the reimaged you to come. And you're going to keep on working the program, keeping yourself in top form into the future. Now, remind yourself you are looking and feeling fabulous these days, and then forget all that for the evening. Eat in a feminine manner, of course, but don't be calculating the calorie content of the entrees on the menu. Don't mention anything about dieting or the like.

My friend Tom said he'd had a lovely dinner date with a woman he'd just met a week earlier at a band concert in the park. The conversation was good, they discovered they shared a number of enthusiasms and opinions. And, Tom said with a smile: "She had a Scotch and soda, a steak, and some concoction called 'chocolate madness' for dessert. Nice for a change to be with a woman who doesn't order white wine and some kind of salad thing."

One more thought about enjoying your dinner: Don't wear your eyeglasses, at least not on your first date or two. Put them on if you must long enough to read the menu, and then put them away. For so many women I have met, the time they first started to need reading glasses was the time they first started feeling old. You don't want to feel old on a date.

LISTEN WELL, TALK WELL...BUT AVOID CERTAIN TOPICS OF CONVERSATION.

This isn't going to be true for all women and all men in all occasions, but generally speaking, a decent man who is just getting to know you does not want to hear about or talk about:
  • your ex-husband or last boyfriend
  • your children's problems
  • his ex-wife or last girlfriend
  • his children's problems

Men find angry, bitter women unattractive. Start discussing the gory details of a previous relationship "gone wrong," and you will lose points.

Try to eliminate nervous chatter, the attempt to fill up silence with talk, any talk.

Years ago, when I was venturing out socially for the first time in over two decades, I met a most attractive man one evening at the restaurant we had agreed upon over the phone. It was the dreaded "blind date!" Arriving a few minutes late, I seemed unable to stop myself from babbling. "I'm a little late," I said, "I'm really sorry. Couldn't get a cab. Never can at this hour, can you? Being a New Yorker, I'm sure you know all about that. You *are* a New Yorker, right? Well, you know what I'm talking about then! Seems like half the cabs vanish off the streets just at the time we need them most...." And on and on I went, unable to stop chattering away, all the while telling myself silently, *Sheila, just shut up! Get a grip on yourself!*

Again, this kind of nervousness gets better over time. It really does. If you fear you're babbling, shift the conversation to him. Remember what your mother told you long ago, that you should ask boys questions about themselves, get them talking about sports or whatever? It's not bad advice with fifty-year-old men either. Most men you'll meet do love talking about themselves, if you are genuinely interested in what they have to say. Also, being a good listener—without fishing for information, without pretending everything he has to say is utterly fascinating—is the best way to learn what this man you're with is really all about, and whether he's someone you'll want to see more of.

And a decent man is also going to be genuinely interested in what you have to say about *you*.

Your reimaged self is not only a woman who looks great; she is an individual with ideas, insights, interests, feelings and experiences of the world. Two human beings can only get to know each other, after all, and develop the trust and understanding that leads to real intimacy, if each has the courage and willingness to be revealing. There's also the matter of basic compatibility: If something you love and enjoy, maybe even dream of as part of your future, happens to be something that turns him off, this is good to know early on.

Here's an example: Judith is a woman who lives in the city, works in the city, but calls herself "a country girl at heart, and I mean deep, deep country!" At the time she met Philip, she was forty-nine, and extremely successful in her own business—so successful that she had already contemplated retiring herself in her early fifties, selling the business, and satisfying her passion "to live with horses and about two dozen dogs." Judith and Philip had a couple of very pleasant evenings out, and discovered common interests and enthusiasms. Horses, dogs and the country life, however, were definitely not among them, which he made crystal clear. If Judith hadn't made her interests known to Philip, she would not have discovered how he felt about them, and that was a piece of information she needed to factor into the picture of any possible relationship.

The point is, sitting back and acting mysterious, or hanging on his every word while offering no words of your own, is wasting time. And you don't have time to waste. Two adults who might actually have a promising future together do not have to have "lots in common," or walk lock-step through life. Each *does* have to get to know what makes the other tick.

One more thing: Don't talk about your age on date one. Try to keep the age thing out of the conversation until you are comfortable with each other. You may find this suggestion offensive, but I believe it's not about being coy—it's just that your reimaged self perhaps looks younger than you are, and men (fools that they are, as we know) prefer younger women, so allow him to preserve the illusion for a bit. If he asks how old you are, simply say, "I never discuss my age. It's just my silly thing." *Don't* ask him to *guess* how old you are. And certainly, don't lie—you'll probably complicate your life. ("Oh what a tangled web we weave," wrote Sir Walter Scott, "when first we practice to deceive!")

Marianne related this experience: "I had been seeing Jim for a couple of months, and I was madly in love. At least I thought I was. We were off to Europe for a week's vacation, and he saw my age on my passport in the airport terminal as we were leaving. I was, in fact, seven years older than I had told him I was. He mentioned this, and said something about how I wasn't too old for him—he just didn't like the fact that I felt I had to lie to him. It was a terribly humiliating experience for me." Marianne decided no more little white lies about her age.

IF YOU TRULY ENJOYED HIS COMPANY AND YOU KNOW HE ENJOYED YOURS, FOLLOW UP ON THAT DELIGHTFUL BEGINNING.

You spent an evening or an afternoon with a new man, you found much about him to admire and like, and you felt quite certain he had an equally enjoyable time with you. Let him know! Men need reassurance about a social success as much as we do.

Tell him that you had a wonderful time. Perhaps you might even try this: Send him flowers. On two very special occasions, with two charming men, I sent flowers to a man at his office on the day following our first date. I enclosed a note saying simply, "Women can do this too! Thank you for a lovely evening. Sheila." Both men loved receiving flowers, and called to tell me so.

After that enjoyable first date, suppose the man you're with asks you out for the following day or evening. If it feels right, go.

After the third or fourth date, offer to make dinner for him. Men really appreciate the home-cooked meal. If your cooking skills are non-existent, splurge on a great bottle of wine, bring in some lovely prepared food, toss out the containers it came in, serve the meal on a pretty table with candles and nice plates. Go for it!

IF YOU'RE UNCERTAIN ABOUT HIS FEELINGS, LET HIM MAKE THE FOLLOW-UP NEXT MOVE.

Perhaps you really liked the man, but you're unsure if he returned your interest. And after the first date, you don't hear from him. Do not call him, even if you really, really want to.

You might wait a month or so, let your feelings and disappointment simmer down, and then give him a call. Have in mind some bit of information or amusing anecdote to tell him, something that relates to an interest of his or to the conversation you had on your date. Then say you hope the two of you will be friends, because you very much enjoyed your evening together. Perhaps you've thought of a woman friend you think he'd be right for; tell him you have a lovely friend he might like to meet. If he says, essentially, thanks but no thanks, let it go. If he says, how nice, he'd like that, tell him a bit about your friend and invite him to one of your "get-togethers."

Suppose you really liked the man, but realize you did or said something that was inappropriate or made him uncomfortable. And he hasn't called. And you're dying to have another shot at him. If by any chance you have a black-tie event coming up in the near future, invite him to be your guest. There's something sort of neutral about the fancy-dress affair (it doesn't seem like a date-date), and for some reason many men will respond positively to such an invitation. Personally, I think they simply enjoy seeing themselves in a tux. Then appear yourself looking drop-dead gorgeous, of course.

The point is this: Compel yourself to read clearly the signals he is giving off. Accept them. A man who has spent some time with you, and who appeared only mildly interested in you, and who makes no move to suggest you see each other again is probably not interested. But you can try to extend the connection (and get a second chance at him) in these couple of ways, without making yourself feel foolish or getting your hopes up.

Nothing ventured, nothing gained.

WHEN IT COMES TO SEX, GO SLOW.

More things your mother told you: A man won't respect you if you go to bed with him too fast.

Actually, what your mother probably said was, he won't respect you if you go to bed with him before you're married. Fortunately, in my opinion, we women no longer are made to feel sex-without-marriage is a bad, bad thing. The first part of that old-fashioned advice, however, does seem to hold true: Men I've talked to in the course of gathering ideas for this book admitted that they lose esteem for a woman who's instantly ready to hop into bed, even if they're delighted to get her there.

Maybe you're very attracted to the new man you have spent the evening with, and you've had a few glasses of wine, and you are definitely turned on and not entirely in control of your actions. Or, after a long dry spell without a man, you are very much in need of confirmation that you're a sexually desirable woman. Or, in your reimaged state you're feeling sexually alluring for the first time in ages, and you're ready for some fun. So you sleep with him.

According to the women I've talked to about this not uncommon situation—and based on my own experiences—nine times out of ten you're going to regret that decision the next day. It's not only that you think he doesn't respect you. *You* don't respect *yourself.*

Sex can be wonderful, with or without marriage—when the man is right and the time is right. For most women, however, sex will be anything but wonderful if it takes place in the absence of a solid and mutual feeling of trust, liking and friendship. The "right man" doesn't have to be a man you know you'd like to spend the rest of your life with. He *does* have to be someone you feel close to, someone with whom you have established at least the beginnings of an emotional connection. He *does* have to be someone you like walking down the street with, holding his arm, talking— and he likes that too. The "right time" doesn't have to mean after two dates or after one month. It *does* have to be after those feelings of trust, liking and friendship have developed.

Some men you'll meet will just want the one-night stand. Trust your gut instincts: If you're listening to them honestly, you'll know. A letch is a letch. If you want to go to bed with a man you suspect is one of those, do so—but don't assume that you're together, that you're in a relationship, or even that you'll hear from him again. In the early stages of your dating, be prepared for making a wrong call or two.

IF YOU WANT A COMMITTED RELATIONSHIP, MAKE YOUR FEELINGS KNOWN.

I'm going out on a limb here, and suggesting that you consider what I'm calling Sheila's three-month action plan. Here it is:

You have been seeing a man for some time. You are quite fond of him and you are certain he is quite fond of you. You have been enjoying a sexual relationship for about three months. Everything is great. *However*, he has expressed no indication that he wants your relationship to turn into a genuinely committed or exclusive one. He may occasionally be seeing other women; you're not sure. Or, you do know that you are the only woman he's involved with, but there are little signs that he's not moving on to the next level: He clams up or gets evasive at any talk of long-range plans, such as where the two of you might take a week's vacation next summer, and so on. And you're wondering where, exactly, you stand. What should you do?

First, I would suggest, proceed with caution. Men tend to get scared really fast! They believe that all women have on their minds is marriage. An exclusive, monogamous relationship sounds to them like a "one step away from the altar" kind of thing, and a man may have various reasons why he's really not ready to think that way. So be careful how you broach the subject.

At the same time, you are absolutely right, in my opinion, to broach it, and to make your wishes known. Remember your goal—to find a wonderful man to share your wonderful self with, for keeps. At this point in your life, you don't want to waste any more time.

So: Make one of your beautiful dinners and put the matter to him, gently. Don't attack him. Don't mention marriage. Don't sound either pleading or resentful. Simply say that you have come to know each other pretty well, you have been sleeping together for three months, you enjoy his company tremendously and you think he enjoys yours. Say that you are interested in a genuinely committed, one-on-one relationship, and if he isn't interested in that as well, he should tell you now.

If he makes it clear (and be prepared for the harsh possibility that he may say so, in so many words) that he does not want or isn't ready for the same thing, move on. Immediately! Not before dinner is over, of course, but in the next days and weeks, begin to separate yourself from him. Yes, you may have to get back out in the single life and go to work again, but you will almost certainly save yourself a lot of grief in the long run.

If the man you are interested in does not wish to see you exclusively, in other words, cut your losses. These years, from age forty to sixty or sixty-five, are crucial to finding that partner, the one you will share the rest of your life with, in sickness and in health and all the rest of it. Don't waste time. The man is not going to change; what you see is what you get. I have known too many women who have devoted their own precious years to men who are never going to commit, who have bided time in relationships that (it was clear almost from the start) weren't going anywhere.

Don't do it. Remind yourself: The man for you is out there. You will find him! Just move on!

WHEN THE TIME IS RIGHT, MENTION MARRIAGE...RIGHT OUT LOUD.

You have moved on to that committed, exclusive relationship. You have been together for a year or more. Everything is great. *However*, you know you want to marry this man, and he's never mentioned marriage. It's time to find out if he's thinking about it, or ever will.

Make another one of your beautiful dinners, and bring up the subject. Why not? Much nicer if he came up with the suggestion first, but remember your goal.

How you talk about marriage will have to do with the nature of your relationship. Said my friend Nancy: "Jack and I always kind of lay our cards on the table with each other. So after we'd been going along so happily for over a year, one evening I said, 'Jack, let's get married. What do you say?'" Jack said, "Okay."

The response you want may not come that easily. If your man gets upset, says he's not that interested in ever getting married, believe him—at least for now. Sometimes a man needs to work his way around to realizing he actually would like to be married, once he's over the shock of the very thought of it. Perhaps you can drop in the information that it's a documented fact that married men live on the average ten years longer than do single men.

If your man says marriage is definitely out of the question, and you know, by the tone of his voice and by all the other clues that have been accumulating, that he's dead serious, believe him. He means it. Then go on with your life in the way that feels right to you—which may be staying in the relationship without the expectation that it will lead to marriage or may be deciding to search elsewhere.

If he says he needs time to think about it all, give it to him. Break up with him if that seems like the right idea, socialize with other men, and let him be alone for a while. A client I worked with did just that, and after six months on his own, her man realized he couldn't live without her.

There are no hard-and-fast rules for all this. You can't force marriage. You must both want the same thing, or it will never work. After a certain age, we all—men and women—come with so much baggage, so much history. Play it by ear—with compassion, kindness and respect for this man you love, but always remembering your own goal, your cause.

NEVER GIVE UP HOPE!

One of my favorite lines of poetry is this, from Emily Dickinson: "Trust in the unexpected." I truly believe that *when you least expect it*, that's when you meet your husband.

My Henry came along when I least expected him to. As I mentioned in the previous chapter, he was the friend of a man I'd talked to at one of my get-togethers. And as I mentioned several chapters ago, I knew almost from the start that I'd found my soul mate. We were married in what our friends said was the most fun, most joyous wedding they'd ever attended. (He wore a tuxedo and—yes!—sneakers.) Henry and I never played games. We both said we were too old and too tired for games. It was right for both of us.

It took me ten years to find him, and a lot of work. But it was my best work. I have a man who loves me and respects me for who I am and for who I am not.

It will happen to you.

A New Challenge: Breast Cancer

I initially intended this book to be a self help for women to change and improve their lives. I wrote it as such, including my life story and how I changed my life at the age forty-three.

I finished this book and felt incredibly excited as I handed it over to my publishers. I had not, however, included any health issues, as it did not seem fitting.

As it would turn out, my life would change only one month before this book was to go to print. I would discover I had breast cancer.

Once again my life would change in ways I had never dreamed possible. I knew I had to write about my experience with this disease as I realized it is very much a part of every woman's life. Any woman can get breast cancer! Any woman can help prevent it! Any woman can fight it and many can beat it! I am, and I will!

The story you are about to read deals with my experiences with this dreadful disease. It is a disease that is the second largest killer of women today. I hope my story will in some way help all my readers to take the preventive measures every woman must make a part of her life to fight this terrible disease.

THE STORY

I had been looking forward to my meeting with my publishers at Paraview for so long. I couldn't wait to discuss when the book would be published, how the cover should be designed, the publicity plans, etc. When the day of the meeting finally came, it started out being the happiest day of my life. Paraview's enthusiasm and support for my book was totally amazing. I couldn't believe it. It was really happening—me, Sheila Grant, an author! All the years of work trying to get this book written and published were really over. After the meeting I left the office and actually skipped down the street like a silly school girl smiling at everyone I saw and actually started to scream out loud with the joy and excitement I felt! Everything seemed perfect.

It seemed that my life was about to take another very dramatic turn now. I would have a book, a website, travel, seminars, television appearances, and much more. The most exciting part of all was that now I finally have the chance to help women everywhere. It was what I had dreamed about for the last fifteen years.

My husband and I had made plans to spend the month of July in France to give us a chance to relax and be together before the book came out. I couldn't wait to leave. Now that all the plans for the book were ready to go, I could really relax. I never thought I could feel so happy, so complete.

I arrived home and immediately called my dearest friend Debra Refson to update her on the book's progress. She is also a writer and had helped me through the long and difficult process of getting this book published. As I blurted out the details of my meeting, I casually looked down at the mail I had brought up with me. I quickly sorted through it while still talking with Debra, and spotted one from the hospital where I had had my yearly mammogram done only a week ago. I opened it while still on the phone, not because I expected any bad news (after all, breast cancer didn't run in my family.) However, as I quickly read the opening statement I knew this was not just the usual routine negative results. It stated that there was a "suspicious" finding and I should call my doctor immediately for further testing.

My heart felt as though it had stopped. I shared my news with Debra who knew from the tone of voice that something was wrong. She told me not to get upset, that it was probably nothing. I asked her how she could say that—Debra had been through breast cancer only five years ago, and I knew how it how changed her life.

I got off the phone and immediately called my close friend and top breast cancer surgeon Dr. Ben Mizrachy. He got right on the phone and told me to calm down. He said it was probably nothing, but I did need to see another radiologist for a second opinion and he suggested one who he worked with and trusted, Dr. Drossman.

I got an appointment for the next day. Ben assured me once again I should not worry. I felt a little better after speaking with him but not much. This was scary stuff!

My two closest friends Debra Refson and Judith Gray insisted on going with me. They tried to keep me laughing and distracted most of the time while waiting to see Dr. Drossman. But as hard as they tried, all I could do was stare at the amazing amount of women in the waiting room! Were they there for the same reason I was? So many of them were young! I thought women didn't have to worry about having a mammogram until they were in their forties. What was going on?

I felt a desperate need to talk to some of them. To my surprise, they were very responsive. It was shocking! Six of the women in the room had or once had breast cancer. Two of the women were in their thirties. Their *thirties*! Each woman started talking about their experiences with cancer. They were all very open and eager to share their stories.

I was feeling more and more confident that I would never be one of these women. I didn't belong there. I wanted to leave. The longer I waited the more I just wanted to get out of there. My friends tried to keep me distracted by trying to make me laugh, but I wasn't in the mood to laugh after hearing all these stories.

Finally it was my turn to see the doctor. She was lovely and immediately started to explain to me what was going to happen. She was going to do a magnification of my breast to see if I needed to have a biopsy. A biopsy? What did she mean by that?

I had the magnifications done and was told to go into another room and wait until the doctor could see me and give me her diagnosis. I sat in that room for the longest forty-five minutes of my life before she reappeared. I knew when she walked into the room that it was not good news.

"Sheila, we will have to do a biopsy immediately. There is a fifty percent chance that this is cancer. I want to schedule this as soon as possible."

I looked at her and started to cry. I'm quite sure she must have to say this quite a few times a day to her patients but she was still very calming and caring. She explained the procedure to me and it sounded very scary. I remember thinking that this simply could not be happening to me. It just couldn't be!

I walked back out into the waiting room, crying hysterically and was very thankful my friends were there. They helped to hold me together while the receptionist scheduled the biopsy for the following Monday. Unfortunately I had to wait out the weekend to get this thing over with.

It would be the longest weekend of my life. All the joy I had felt was gone. All I could think about was the fact that I might have cancer. My husband and I were scheduled to leave for France in just nine days. I wished I had never gone for the stupid mammogram or at least waited until I got back from my vacation.

Monday came and I had the biopsy which turned out to be far more difficult and frightening than I had been prepared for. They placed me face down on a table with my one breast exposed through a hole in the table and the doctor went in with a huge needle and probe and extracted quite a lot of tissue from my breast. It was not pleasant, to say the least. It was far more upsetting and painful than I had expected. It took almost two hours. My husband was with me and took me home trembling like a very frightened child. I would not know the results for two full days, maybe three.

I had no idea how I would be able to wait for three days for the results. I was feeling so frightened, so scared, so angry at myself for not feeling strong.

The phone rang the next afternoon and I heard Dr. Drossman's voice. I knew the answer already. She minced no words, got straight to the point. I had cancer and would have to have surgery right away. She wished me luck and said not to worry; the good news was that it was in it's earliest stage and I would not lose my whole breast.

I got off the phone and cried until there were no more tears. The phone rang again. I picked it up, still sobbing, and somehow managed a "hello". It was Ben.

"Sheila, I just spoke with Dr. Drossman. I am so sorry but please know that you are a very lucky woman. You are going to be fine. The cancer is in its earliest stages, but we do need to operate right away. I was supposed to leave for vacation tomorrow but I just canceled my trip. I have scheduled surgery for tomorrow morning. Let's get this thing over with and I believe you will still be able to leave Saturday for France. We will do it! We'll get you cancer free then you will go away and relax with Henry. You'll unfortunately need to have two months of radiation when you come back, but we will talk about that tonight in my office. I want you and Henry to come to my office at 10:00 tonight to go over all the details. You are to go over to the hospital this afternoon for blood work."

"Ben, please tell me the truth," I said, between sobs. "Am I going to die? I really want to know right now. I have to know right this minute. Am I dying?"

"Of course not, Sheila," he said sympathetically. "Have you not been hearing what I've said? You are going to be absolutely fine! Now I know all of this is a shock to you and that it's a lot to take in all at once, but I will explain everything to you and Henry tonight. You will be perfect again and cancer free after the surgery and radiation. You have to trust me. I would not lie to you."

"You are sure, Ben?" I asked. "You promise there isn't something you aren't telling me?"

"I promise" he said. "And you are still going to France!"

Henry and I arrived at Ben's office that night at 9:45. The office still had three women waiting to see him. Why? Why are so many women getting breast cancer? Something far greater than I had ever imagined was showing its ugly face. Something that I had thought only happened to other women—namely, older women— was happening to young and old alike. Something far bigger and more onerous than anything I could have imagined. And now I was one of those women who had probably all said the same thing I did: It could never happen to me!

I had dozens of questions for Ben and so did Henry. He was extremely patient and careful to answer every question with absolute honesty and candor. I asked him if he worked every night to 11:00 taking new patients. He smiled sadly and confessed that it happened more often than he'd like.

I trusted this man. I trusted him with my life. One of the finest surgeons in the country, people fly from all over the world to get

Ben's opinion and help. I didn't need a second opinion. After one hour of discussion I said, "I think we better get home so we can all grab a few hours of sleep." I turned to Ben. "After all, I need you feeling rested to operate on me tomorrow. Let's get this over with."

The operation went as scheduled the following morning. Henry, Debra, Judith were all there for me—for more hours than I think they counted on. Between the operation and recovery room time, I was not to see them for about six hours.

Ben was there as I opened my eyes after the operation wearing the biggest smile I ever saw. "Everything went absolutely perfectly! I think we got all of it and I am even more optimistic than ever that you are going to be just fine!"

I paled. "What do you mean, you *think* you got all of it. I don't understand? You mean I may still have cancer?"

"Well Sheila, we do have to wait for the pathology report to see if the margins are clear. They most likely are, but with your particular type of cancer it had to be done a little differently and will take another two days or so to be completely sure. Don't worry—this is a standard procedure. I did have to make a bigger incision than I had thought, as we did have to take quite a bit of tissue out. I have a rather large bandage on you now. But I think it will heal well."

I was shocked. "Why didn't you tell me any of this last night? You said I would have a small incision and shouldn't be a big deal. Now you say I still may have some cancer left and you had to make a large incision. I don't understand. What are you trying to tell me, Ben?" I started to cry. My body became very, very cold and was shaking uncontrollably.

"Sheila, I did tell you and Henry that the tissue I took would have to go to the pathologist. That is standard procedure. As for the size of the incision it is a bit larger than I had anticipated but no doctor can tell you exactly how large it will be until they go in. I feel quite sure that you are going to heal beautifully and I would not let myself worry about that now. I wanted to make sure I got it all and left you with clean margins."

Henry took me home, and although I finally calmed down and stopped shaking, I became very depressed. I thought I would feel better once the surgery was over but I certainly didn't. I arrived home and climbed into my bed exhausted from the day and didn't want to speak to anyone. Henry didn't know what to do. I took a big long look at the huge bandage over my breast wondering what my breast really looked like. I thought about having to wait for another pathology report and decided to take a valium, pull the covers over my head and go to sleep.

The next morning I awoke and knew I had to force myself out of this slump. I looked in the mirror and said "Sheila Grant, you are acting like a child. You are going to be fine. You've been through a lot in your life and have survived it all. You are a strong woman. Remember that! Go read your book!"

I managed to actually start to feel a little better and started to prepare myself for the trip, pulling clothes from the closet and making lists of what I would need to take with me. I was going on that trip! Nothing would stop me. Nothing!

However, the next day I got another phone call from Ben. "Sheila, I have some bad news. We need to go back in and remove some more tissue. The margins didn't come back clean. Now, do not worry, this often happens and it is very difficult to know until the pathologist report comes back. Now, I suggest we do the surgery on Friday morning and get this over with. I will be going back in the same incision and just removing a bit more tissue. If all goes well, I will still let you and Henry leave Saturday night for France, believe it or not!"

I just said, "Okay, Ben. Friday morning." I couldn't say anything else to him. What else was there to say? I still had cancer in my body and I knew that I would have to be foolish to say, "Well Ben, I won't let you go back in. I am going to keep this cancer with me until I get back from France."

The surgery went as smoothly as it did the first time. My bandage was larger this time and that immediately upset me. Ben said it was to protect me from infection. I was sent home, and Ben said if I felt well enough that I could leave the next night for France. I needed rest now and that seemed like a perfect place. I was to take it extremely easy and relax. Sure

Henry and I actually did manage to leave that next night. I don't know how we did it—I was so depressed and feeling so tired, that I was barely able to walk. The wheel chair got me on the plane and off, which made me feel very old, very tired and very sad. I kept thinking that my poor husband had a mutilated wife now. But I had no idea what my breast really looked like under that giant bandage.

A couple of weeks later, I found out. I removed the bandage, and stood in front of the mirror. I almost fainted! I had less than two thirds of my breast left. It was horrible. I cried and cried and cried. I decided to cover it right back up. I never wanted Henry to see me like this. I thought it would make him sick. It made *me* sick! I never imagined in a million years it would look so hideous. All sorts of thoughts ran through my head: Henry would never be able to make love to me again, he would he leave me, my life would never be normal again.

When I got back to the U.S., I realized that cancer had already changed my life. What I had to do was to find out why, and how I could get my life back. I had so much to look forward to: my book, my family, my wonderful friends. I had so many blessings. I had to learn to understand and deal with all my emotions, and not let this disease get the best of me.

I decided to add my story to this book, because the harsh truth is that any woman can get cancer. But I believe that any woman can also beat it. *I* will beat it! Women and the doctors in this country will have to change their old way of thinking. We must start insisting that women even in their twenties do self examinations and possibly have mammograms if there are any suspicious findings.

I started radiation last week. It isn't as terrible as I expected. I addressed my mutilated breast with three doctors who all say I can have reconstruction in seven to eight months. Until then Henry only gets to see one breast when we make love. I have invented an outrageous bra that works quite well for this problem. I know now that Henry couldn't care less what my breast looks like. He loves me—the whole me—and I know and believe that with all my heart.

I have met and spoken to so many women sitting in the various doctor's offices and have learned so much. Breast cancer kills so many women, young and old alike. It leaves women feeling devastated, alone, vulnerable, un-whole. Most breast cancer survivors say they will never feel the same again, their life was changed forever by cancer.

As difficult as this experience was, I am getting stronger every day. I can beat this. Any woman can. Now I intend to put a great deal of my time and effort into helping other women with breast cancer get through it and understand what is going on. I want to make people aware that cancer has no face or color or age. Knowledge is the key here. Women everywhere must understand the facts and the warning signs early enough to take action before the cancer does. It doesn't have to run in your family, as many people believe. Only one third of cancer victims have a family history of it.

All women, regardless of their age, should do self examinations regularly. A mammogram should be scheduled immediately if there are any suspicious findings at all. The women I see going through radiation and chemotherapy are in their twenties, thirties, forties, all the way to their eighties.

I just found out a most shocking fact last week. I had this cancer three years ago! I had breast reduction and the mammogram I was required to take showed that there were suspicious findings. I needed magnifications and a biopsy before my surgery. I was sent for a second opinion to a top radiologist who gave me a sonogram and said I was fine and to go on and have my surgery.

What I didn't know and the radiologist should have known was that a sonogram could never have found my cancer. Only the suggested magnifications and biopsy could have. Unfortunately, my plastic surgeon was never told by his secretary that I had this problem. He should never have operated on me. I believe it was up to him to have looked at all my records before operating, not to leave such an important matter up to a secretary. But it is too late now.

My reason for telling you about this incident is that women have to go for two or even three opinions if there is any doubt about the diagnosis. I fell through the cracks. All of this could have been avoided three years ago. I have become extremely angry since seeing all my former reports. This should never have happened. Never! I have lost part of my breast now and have suffered severe depression all because of a misdiagnosis and a top surgeon's neglect.

My dear friend Debra, who is extremely spiritual, said to me soon after my surgery, "Sheila, I know you will never believe me now or understand what I am going to say, but I believe there was a reason you got breast cancer. I don't know the reason now and I don't know when or how but I believe you will realize this and it will change your life in some positive way. I know it has changed my life in so many positive ways." Debra is a cancer survivor of eight years.

I had no idea what she was talking about then. Her words only irritated me and made me angrier than I already was. I was going to be happy to have experienced cancer? Not a chance!

It has taken me quite awhile, but only now have I started to understand what she meant. My breast cancer was diagnosed at this time of my life—just as my book will be coming out—just when I can get my word out to thousands of women about what happened to me, and how it could have been avoided. I am being given an opportunity to help other women who might be able to benefit from my story and take the preventative measures to help themselves avoid this awful disease.

I have set up a section on my website about cancer, which takes my reader through all the stages of my recovery and gives weekly updates as to what happens to me. I will also be giving the most up-to-date advice from the country's top specialists on the subject. I am very excited about this project and have started to feel very optimistic about my life once again. Any Woman Can!

APPENDICES:
Advice from the Experts

Teeth

by Dr. Michael Kraus

Have you ever been to a cocktail party and seen a well-dressed, striking individual you just *had* to meet? You meander your way over and finally muster the nerve to introduce yourself. But when he or she opens his or her mouth to smile, suddenly the entire fabulous package falls apart! Why? Because the mouth and teeth are a virtual disaster area. I'm not simply referring to the sushi caught between the two central incisors, but to teeth which are chipped, misaligned, or noticeably yellowed. Indeed, even a seemingly flawless package can suddenly be ruined by a set of bad teeth. Could this be true about people's first impression of you?

Your mouth, teeth and overall smile are so important to a first impression. People read into what they see in a person's mouth: she's happy, she's sad, she's excited, she's embarrassed, she's angry, she's lying. Worse yet, she looks like a horse, a beaver, a rodent, a hillbilly. Perfect teeth go hand in hand with the new image you have worked so hard to create. People in high position or visibility scream with incongruity without wonderful teeth. Thus, the next step on our journey to maximize your image potential lies with the enhancement or creation of a dynamic and beautiful smile. When a patient takes that step to have her teeth redone, she can be transformed so dramatically that her entire face will brighten and regain its vivacity and youth. In a social environment, whether on a date or with friends, an individual's comfort or confidence can be aided or even defined by her smile. A dynamic smile in the work place will open doors you did not know existed. Only a perfect set of teeth will give you the confidence you require.

If you are like most people, the concept of having your teeth done terrifies you. But the fact is, redoing one's teeth need not be a painful or lengthy process. Dentists equipped with the most advanced technology use lasers and drills to achieve almost instant results with minimal discomfort. Imagine for example that your dark, stained teeth can be leaser-bleached in a period of three hours, while a more involved procedure such as porcelain veneers can be completed in just a few days' time. Many patients who were reluctant to go through a long and painful dental overhaul now have little excuse in delaying reconstruction procedures.

It is crucial, however, to have the right person guide you through this process. There are many looks available to the patient. It is important to keep in mind that what may appear to be a perfect set of teeth on one person would be a disaster in another's mouth. Large beautiful teeth framed in a large joker-like smile will look like a set of chiclets in a small mouth. Small symmetrical teeth in a diminutive mouth look right. However, those same teeth in a large mouth will look lost and show large, dark voids.

Whatever the case, it is much easier and less expensive to change the teeth and gums rather than the lips. An excellent dentist will determine what suits his patient best. Your imager will be able to direct you to the best dentists who will use both their talents and imagination to determine what look is right for you.

The mouth and teeth can give a person an impression that is a lasting image. Not only are they a tip off to the emotions of the minute, but they can reveal clues to a person's character and upbringing as well, be it true or false. Badly chipped or misaligned teeth give the appearance of a lazy person. To some, it may be representative of class or privilege. And buck teeth can give the appearance of stupidity, while a protruding jaw, the unattractive Cro-Magnon appearance. A bad orthodontic job (braces) can thin out what was once a voluptuous full upper lip by bringing the teeth too far in.

I have a patient who is a news anchor woman and had just come to me after having had her teeth done (twenty-four of them). She got her head shots back and she thought she looked terrible. True, her teeth were brand new and bright as day, but they looked awful. To boot, she was recently divorced and had begun dating again and felt even worse than she did before having her teeth done. She looked like she was wearing a bad set of dentures. What was the problem? The dentist had followed her lip line when creating her smile, which unfortunately slanted up to the left. Her entire upper and lower teeth were done at an angle! We redid her entire mouth at the proper angle—parallel to her eyes, not her lips—and the results were fabulous.

All of the above form a subliminal picture which is either pleasing or quite possibly repelling. I am not saying that it is fair or that people are shallow enough to believe their initial impressions are representative of people's personalities, but these impressions cannot be ignored. If what you seek is a new, improved image, your teeth may very well be the crucial ingredient needed to change your appearance enough to deliver the new you. The wonderful thing about a great smile is that it will actually become even more radiant and more attractive the more you use it. The good news is, it is relatively easy to transform a less than attractive smile into a fabulous one. Why not match the inner you with a warm, brilliant smile, one that will enhance your facial expressions and give renewed youth to your appearance?

If you have decided it is time to work on your teeth, it is either for cosmetic reasons or physiological ones:

PHYSIOLOGICAL

1. Your teeth are killing you! Pain is not going to encourage you to smile prettily at a party.
2. Your gums bleed all the time.
3. Your bad breath is slaying all potential dates.
4. When you speak, spittle comes through the large open spaces between your teeth.
5. When you eat, food gets caught between your teeth.
6. You speak with a lisp.

COSMETIC

1. Your teeth have many spaces, cracks, or are misshapen.
2. Dark color or stains.
3. Overly long teeth.
4. Overly large gums.
5. Overly short teeth.
6. Overlapping teeth
7. "Fake-looking" teeth.

Whether physiological or cosmetic, your reasons are valid. And if your reason(s) are in the above list, there *is* something you can do about it!

Thin or Missing Upper Lip

A beautiful, fifty-year-old woman came into my office complaining that now that her orthodontics was complete and her teeth were straight, she needed the name of a plastic surgeon to plump her lip up. After all, we all want voluptuous lips, don't we? After examining her, it was obvious that her teeth now offered her no support for her upper lip. I call it the "de-feminization of the American Woman" by orthodontists. In a patient's quest to straighten or correct her bite, the patient's profile was never considered. By removing all of a person's bicuspids, the lip has nothing to do but fall! We fixed this problem by performing a "lip lift" without plastic surgery. I merely changed the position of her upper teeth by pushing the edges out ever so slightly.

But watch out: the opposite can also be the case when teeth are so large they stretch the lip to the point of thinning it. In this case, you end up looking like your lips simply won't cover your teeth, which isn't very attractive either.

Gums That Just Don't Quit

No matter how perfect your teeth are, if you have an overly large gum area, that is all people will see. And if you have ugly teeth and vast wastelands of gum tissue it will completely steal the beauty from your face and the wonderful image you have thus far achieved.

When a patient presents a gummy smile, we must evaluate carefully, and sometimes take aggressive measures in order to achieve a wonderful smile. Gum tissue may need to be removed surgically or by laser in order to move the gum line upward. Sometimes bone must be removed as well.

This procedure may be a little less instantaneous than you would like but beware of the dentist who says that he can cure your overly-large gums in three days with only porcelain laminates. Surgery means you may need to go through some effort and discomfort, but the results are dramatic, and definitely worth it.

Dark Teeth or Opaque Crowns

There is simply no excuse for dark teeth with the advent of laser bleaching, porcelain laminates (veneers) and porcelain jackets. And because whitening is so available, the woman with dark teeth has little excuse. Laser bleaching, however, is not for everyone. It does not work on crowns, and some people are highly sensitive to the procedure.

But don't despair! Porcelain laminates, when done properly, are totally natural-looking and do not fade in color like bleaching. Your new image demands white teeth and the wonderful part of veneers is that they feel exactly like your own teeth. Have you ever seen someone with dark rings around every tooth? The metal edges of the crowns are showing, or the crowns have either stained the gums, or stained the teeth. Another common problem are blocky "opaque chiclet" teeth. With new all-ceramic crowns, it is easy to replace them with natural looking translucent teeth.

Bad Breath

Last of all, and perhaps most important, a little something about bad breath. If you have bad breath, you are not attractive to anyone. Do something about it! People *do* notice. Believe it or not, halitosis *is* a cosmetic issue and if you wish to present or re-present yourself to the world it can be a handicap.

Bad breath is caused by one or more of the following:

1) Bad dentistry or tooth decay.

2) Periodontal or gum disease.

3) Systemic (body) issues.

4) Smoking and coffee.

Eliminating some bad habits and redoing old dentistry will usually cure the problem. In my office there are also prescriptive kits to help remedy the problem.

The key to successful dental treatment is that it is dramatic yet undetectable. Perfect teeth that are noticeably false strike a bad chord. Chiclet-white upper teeth with lower cigarette-stained teeth do not work. A perfect set of twenty visible teeth are drowned out by two inches of gum on top or dark voids to each side. That is not to say that perfect is always correct. Variance can be what makes one's smile perfectly natural. That is always my goal and should be that of the cosmetic dentist you choose. What is best for the patient? With your input he or she should know what's right for you.

Dr. Michael Kraus has been practicing general and cosmetic dentistry for the past 17 years in New York City. He has appeared on numerous television and radio shows on topics ranging from laser dentistry to porcelain laminates. Dr. Kraus has represented Premier Laser and ADT Laser at the Greater New York Dental Meeting and he lectures throughout the country. He is also an instructor with Aesthetic Advantage, a program which focuses on porcelain laminate dentistry.

APPENDIX B

Skin

by Dr. Howard Sobel

Here are the latest procedures for the skin.

Botox Treatments

This is a simple procedure that's considered safe. It takes only five minutes and requires no recovery time. Using a micro-sized needle, Botox is injected into certain muscles in the face and neck to relax them and lessen the appearance of wrinkles that result from our daily expressions such as crow's feet, worry lines, frown lines and laugh lines. This is an effective means of reversing the visible signs of aging. The results can be seen within four days and last 3-6 months, depending on the individual.

Collagen-Hylaform-Dermalogen

Facial lines, wrinkles, nasolabial folds, lips and depressed scars can now be instantly smoothed, softened and plumped. This safe, non-surgical treatment replaces the natural collagen support layer underneath the skin, with results lasting 3-6 months. Allergy testing may be required four weeks prior to initial treatment.

Autologous-Fat Transfers

Autologous treatments use the patient's own body fat to plump up facial hollowness, and fill in facial lines and wrinkles. This procedure lasts longer than collagen, is non-allergenic, and yields almost instantaneous results, some of which are permanent.

Soft Form-Alloderm

This is available as a permanent filler treatment, best recommended for lips or nasolabial folds.

Glycolic Acid-TCA Facial Treatments

Bring back the glow of healthy skin or minimize hyperpigmented areas using increasing strengths of pure alpha-hydroxy acid or TCA. This treatment will remove outer layers of dead cells, encouraging cell renewal and revealing fresher, younger skin. This peel is most effective using a series of six, applied in two week intervals. Recommended for most skin types, especially mature, dull and sun-damaged skin. Also used as part of an acne care regimen.

Refinity (70) glycolic acid) Treatment

This intense peel uses higher concentrations of alpha-hydroxy acid combined with a unique anti-inflammatory agent to deliver a rapid exfoliation of the top layers of skin without redness or discomfort. A perfect procedure for refining fine lines and lightening pigmentation from age, sun and pregnancy. A Refinity peel can be repeated every two weeks and is performed by one of our specially trained cosmetic nurses.

Jessner's—TCA Peel

This peel combines Trichloracetic Acid (TCA) with Jessner's solution, which contains several potent exfoliating agents including

Resorcinol, salicyclic and lactic acid, which penetrates deeper into skin to clear stubborn acne, scaring, hyperpigmentation and deeper wrinkling. Patients can expect to peel for five to seven days. Consultation and pretreatment are required.

Microdermabrasion

Microdermabrasion is a non-invasive, non-surgical procedure that uses a highly controlled spray of organic mineral crystals. This treatment removes the outer layer of damaged skin, revealing younger, tighter and more radiant skin below the surface. Face, hands and décolleté will benefit from this effective treatment. May be used in conjunction with our Non-Ablative lasers for synergistic results. Performed by our highly trained estheticians or cosmetically trained nurses.

LASER TREATMENTS

Pigmented Lesions—Sun Damage and Tattoos

An FDA approved state of the industry laser quickly lightens and removes age spots in addition to other brown discolorations of the face, hands and body. It is also effective in the removal of tattoos.

Fine Lines and Wrinkles

The Erbium, CO2 Coblation or Non-Ablative lasers resurface fine lines and wrinkles for a more youthful appearance. The cool touch II laser is a less aggressive treatment for patients who must return to their regular activities quickly. Cool touch II facial rejuvenation was designed to combat the effects of aging in a softer, gentler way. It uses a revolutionary process that delivers the laser energy through your skin's surface to gently stimulate the production of collagen, while protecting the outer layer of your skin, with no down time.

Telangiectasia Dilated-Blood Vessels

Using the Versapulse C Laser, as well as many other lasers, we can instantaneously remove small, unsightly blood vessels located on the face and legs. There is no bruising or down time associated with this procedure.

Laser Hair Removal

The Light Sheer Diode Laser is the most successful technique available for removing unwanted hair, resulting in an 80% permanent hair reduction. Hair can quickly be removed from the face, neck, abdomen, breasts, arms, underarms, bikini line, back, shoulders, chest, ears, and between the eyebrows with little or no discomfort.

BODY TREATMENTS

Spider Vein Treatment

This non-surgical procedure can rid the skin of unsightly veins. A sclerosing solution is injected into the vein, causing it to shrink and eventually disappear.

Body Contouring-Liposuction

This surgical technique permanently removes fat cells in the stubborn areas that dieting and exercise don't help. A pioneer of this surgery, Dr.Sobel has safely and successfully performed over 2000 liposuctions since 1986 using the tumescent procedure under local anesthesia. This technique, in conjunction with the power assisted cannula, results in less bruising, less swelling and better skin contraction. Surgery is performed in our in-house, accredited operating rooms.

COSMETIC TREATMENTS

Wax

Get rid of unwanted facial hair using an exclusive natural European wax infused with essential oils and Vitamin E. Available for the lip, chin, eyebrow or full face. Suitable for all skin types, especially sensitive skin.

Eye Lash and Eyebrow Tinting

Great for fair-haired people who want their eyelashes and eyebrows to stand out, or for those who just want a more natural but defined eye. A replacement for daily mascara or eyebrow pencil application using a safe and non-toxic dye to enhance eyes.

Permanent Makeup

Natural pigments are applied through a special handpiece. Using new micropigmentation techniques, eyebrows can be recreated using fine lines to simulate real hair, soft eyeliners can enhance the eyes and lip liner can create a fuller lip. Great for women with thin or no eyebrows, who are allergic to cosmetics, who workout a lot, sufferers of alopecia, or poor eyesight, and busy women who are short on time.

HAIR TRANSPLANTATION

Using the new micro and mini graft technique, we successfully transplant hair to bald areas. The fact that surgery was performed will be nearly undetectable.

Dr. Howard Sobel received his degree in medicine from the Albert Einstein School of Medicine and completed his residency in dermatology and dermatology and dermatologic surgery at Emory University School of Medicine. He is board Certified in Dermatological and Cosmetic Surgery, as well as being the editor in chief of the International Journal of Cosmetic Surgery and Aesthetic Dermatology. He has appeared on major television network programs and has been featured in such publications as Vogue, Elle, Marie Claire, Allure and Cosmopolitan. Dr. Sobel helped to pioneer the union of dermatology with cosmetic surgery. He was among the first surgeons to perform liposuction using the tumescent solution purely under local anesthesia. He has also had over twenty years of experience in effectively treating all skin related conditions including cancer etc.

Cosmetic Surgery

By Robert M. Freund, M.D., FACS

Cosmetic surgery, once deemed only a privilege of the rich and famous, now has become more popular than ever. Newer, safer techniques and increased availability have brought surgery for the sake of personal improvement into the mainstream. As a result of the increased demand for cosmetic procedures, the techniques have improved in one particular area at the cost of unsightly scars or other unacceptable sequella. Furthermore, today's techniques focus a significant amount of attention on recreating the ideal feminine contour. Natural results, avoiding the "done" look are now an achievable goal! What can you as the consumer look forward to?

The aging face suffers from several key problems that have had new techniques created in the recent past to slow the clock of time while maintaining the subtle, refreshed look.

Eyebrows/Eyelids

The eyebrows and eyelids tend to show signs of age and gravity in the patient's early forties. As the eyebrows sag, the forehead wrinkles while straining to maintain eyebrow height. Despite the increased exertion to hold up the eyebrow, the sagging results in increased heaviness and extra skin on the upper eyelids. The lower lids also show signs of aging with bags and excess skin. Older techniques focus on grossly elevating the eyebrow, forsaking the natural arched shape of the eyebrow. This creates a surprised look and typically elevates the hairline too high. My technique of integrating a limited lateral brow lift with eyelid rejuvenation creates a gracefully arched eyebrow with a youthful upper eyelid. At the same time, the hairline is left intact and the small patch of thinning hair in the temples is removed. The technique also improves the lower eyelid by removing skin and bulging fat from inside the eyelid. Finally, external scars are eliminated and a more natural eyelid contour is produced.

Face

The midface or cheek region often droops in middle-aged females, yielding a tired hollow appearance to the region below the eyes. Up to now, little has been done to address this problem. However, new techniques elevate the cheeks with small incisions placed in the temples. This technique can be combined with other limited scar techniques around the face to yield subtle improvements that yield a refreshed look.

The lower face including the jowls and neck has been given much attention lately in plastic surgery circles. Although the actual technique to tighten these regions and the desired look has not changed, recently limited scar techniques have been introduced. These techniques place the majority of scar behind the ears in a limited fashion. For patients with short, closely cropped hair, or for those who like to wear their hair back, this is a quantum leap forward, allowing them to stay younger looking without having to sacrifice their hair style.

Breasts

Breast surgery has had the greatest improvement in techniques and results in the recent past. The breast is composed of a skin envelope, breast tissue and fat. Blood vessels and nerves course through the breast to provide sensation and oxygen to the breast. The female breast after pregnancy undergoes several changes. The skin stretches and sags. The breast tissue also stretches and loses its shape as well as volume. In the past, breast lifts and breast reductions were based on the removal of a large amount of the skin envelope to create the desired shape for the breast. However, this technique suffers from several major design flaws. Firstly, the tension created by tightly draping a reduced skin envelope around a sagging breast will cause the skin to stretch and sag in less than a year. Furthermore, the tension created by reducing the envelope leads to disfiguring widened scars. Finally, no attempt was made to create a natural tear-drop shaped breast, like the one mother nature intended women to have.

Today, breast reduction surgery can be performed through limited incisions, either around the nipple or down the breast (not the "anchor scar" of old). The main ingredient of the new techniques is liposuction of the breast tissue to enhance the longevity of the breast shaping, and to limit the size change with weight loss or weight gain. After the liposuction, the breast tissue is shaped to create an appealing breast contour. Thus any redraping of the skin is done with minimal tension, and scars heal to an almost invisible line. This technique can be combined with breast implants for those patients desiring a breast lift with an enlargement . Be careful of doctors advising breast implants alone to correct loss of breast volume and sagging combined. This technique usually results in the larger than desired breasts that continue to sag creating the "rock in a sock" look.

Body contouring requires evaluation of the skin elasticity and quality, fat distribution and contour as well as the underlying muscle integrity. Those doctors who provide liposuction to their patients should be able to evaluate and treat shortcomings in all of these structures. When considering body contour surgery, as with all other cosmetic surgery, as with all other cosmetic surgery, proportion and aesthetic ideal are important. When more than liposuction is needed, as when excess skin is present on the abdomen or thighs, or when the muscles of the abdomen are weakened as a result of pregnancy or previous surgery, newer techniques focus on recreating the feminine abdominal contour with excellent scarring. This new technique is known as the high lateral tension abdomenoplasty.

Finally, choosing a plastic surgeon to perform your surgery can be a daunting task. Of course, you will only go to a board-certified plastic surgeon that has been referred to you by a close friend. But, once you interview a plastic surgeon to perform your surgery, listen to his/her advice. If the advice does not sound right to you, it probably isn't. Also, ask to see photos of patients with similar problems to yours. If they are acceptable, then ask if you could speak to some of them about their experience with the procedure. Do your homework and you will increase your chances of an excellent outcome.

Robert M. Freund, M.D., FACS is a board-certified plastic surgeon practicing in Manhattan.

Vocal Image

By Lucille S. Rubin, Ph.D.

My phone rings. Each caller has a different story to tell:

"My voice mail really doesn't sound like me."

"My boss says my voice is hard on his ears."

"Just because I work with men, I don't think I have to sound like one."

"My best friend tells me I always sound as if I'm whining."

"I'm tired of people saying, 'what did you say?'"

"I know I'm good at what I do, but nobody listens to me in the meetings."

"My last performance review said my voice gets high when I get emotional."

"Sometimes I feel as if I have marbles in my mouth."

"My friends say I talk too fast for them to follow what I'm saying."

"I'm smart, but my voice sounds ditsy."

"My strong voice works in the court room, but not in the bedroom."

"At social engagements, people always ask me where I'm from."

"Ahhh, hummmm, my last interview... uhmmmm... was a disaster."

"I'm the boss, but I'm told I sound too tough and aggressive."

"I'm twenty-seven years old and my voice sounds as if I'm fifteen!"

"I have to talk all day on the job, and my voice gets tired and raspy."

"I think my dates think I'm a pushover because I have a breathy voice."

"I'm scared to death to speak in front of others."

"I'm told that my voice is monotone."

"My tongue is not in the right place for my S's; They sound too hissy."

"People listen to my accent more than to what I'm saying."

These representative complaints come from people who phone my studio every day to express their frustrations. Some of the concerns deal with vocal tone while others point to articulation problems or accent reduction. The remedy is to change their vocal image. "But can I change my voice and the way I speak?" is the usual follow-up question. The answer is yes, you can—and in many different ways.

First, it's important to understand your voice, its potential and how it can better serve your personal and professional life. Whether you want to find a boyfriend, ace the interview, engage your listener, persuade your spouse, get your kids to behave, keep your cool, comfort a friend, manage the team, or turn on a lover, you'll want to send a clear message wrapped up in a warm and winning voice and delivered with your best speaking skills.

Hear Your voice as Others Do

If you've listened to your outgoing phone message or heard your voice on tape, you've probably remarked as one of the callers above: "I don't think I really sound like that." Maybe your phone and tape recorder aren't state of the art, but the sound on the tape is very similar to that which your listeners hear.

We hear our voices through sound waves and through bone conduction, but our listeners hear our voices only through sound waves. Because we hear differently, our perceptions differ. So, if you want others to listen to you, you had best adjust your voice and make it appealing to their ears.

If you're willing to change your voice, you've already started to find a new vocal image. You can make subtle changes every day if you are clear about the way you want to be perceived: weak or strong, shy or confident, clear or confused. You are in charge of how you want to sound.

TIP: *Read aloud three minutes a day. Tape, replay and assess your voice by describing what you like about it and what you'd like to change. Encourage your next reading to use more of the vocal choices you like.*

Posture affects your voice

Susan, one of the distressed callers, came into my studio to rehearse a presentation she had to give the next day to a client. She was nervous about how she would perform, so I suggested I role-play the client. She started to talk and within one minute I let my head nod and a snore escape. She got my point. We moved to a full-length mirror where she saw her slumped spine and rounded shoulders. Next, I played back one minute of her presentation and Susan heard her unenthusiastic voice. We immediately began work on aligning her body to find a positive statement. I encouraged her to lengthen her spine, open her chest and balance her body weights. These changes, much to her surprise, also affected the sound of her voice.

Good posture frees the breath, releases body tensions and encourages an aligned vocal tract. Susan put all of this to work for her overnight. She called the next day after the presentation to say she had gotten the contract. "What do you think helped you the most?" I asked.

"You turned my head around," she said. "When I felt the power of my body and the strength of my personal presence, this big voice came out of me! I knew I was in control."

TIP: *Imagine your vertebrae as children's blocks and stack them up for a long spine. Open your chest by sliding your shoulder blades together. Balance your three heavy weights by placing your head over your shoulders, and your shoulders over your pelvis. Avoid leading with your head, crumpling your chest and slumping your spine.*

Vocal Production

Knowing how your voice works gives you a handle on changing your vocal image. Here are the four steps in the vocal process: First, air flows in (respiration); Second, the air brings the vocal folds together and creates voice (phonation); Third, the voice travels through the vocal tract on up into the cavities of the head (resonation); Fourth, the voice is shaped into vowels and consonants by the jaw, tongue, palate and lips (articulation). It's exciting to know that this process works beautifully if we allow nature to do its work. The voice tends to get into trouble when we manipulate our breath, push or hold back our voice, favor one resonator (for example, our nose) and are careless about engaging our articulators. Change any of the four steps in vocal production and you will affect a change in your vocal image.

Eight Ways to Change Your Vocal Image

You can project a positive vocal image by optimizing the way you breathe, phonate, resonate and articulate. Further, you can alter people's perception of your voice by finding an appealing quality and using variety in volume, rate and pitch.

The tips and exercises offered below will develop your awareness, but reaching your goals may take professional coaching. Be ready to apply these options by speaking your outgoing voice mail message or reading aloud from the newspaper or from a poem.

1. Breathe from your belly: Place your hand over your navel and breathe. You should feel your belly float out as you inhale and feel your belly float in as you exhale. Avoid chest activity and raising your shoulders by looking in a full-length mirror. Speak using belly breathing for achieving full voice.

2. Keep your throat open: Pinch your nostrils closed and open your mouth. Get used to breathing in and out of your mouth. Open your mouth, relax the back of your tongue and yawn up the back of your throat (palate.) Release your nostrils and keep the awareness of the space at the back of your throat. Speak and feel the air flowing through your throat. Use the open throat sensation for free and relaxed sound.

3. Mix your resonators: Place one hand on your forehead and the other on your chest bone. Hum a sustained note, sensing vibrations on your forehead. Next, drop your jaw and say "ah" as if a doctor were looking down your throat. Be aware of the vibrations in your chest. Finally, on one breath, hum into the dropped jaw position on "ah" and go into "um" maintaining chest vibrations. Practice speaking with an equal mix of chest and head vibrations.

In my coaching practice, I've found that many women lack

chest resonance; however, if your voice is dark and heavy, you'll want more top vibrations. Remember to blend both top and bottom (chest and head) much like the mix of the tweeter and woofer on your stereo.

4. *Activate your articulators*: jaw, tongue, palate, and lips.

a. Jaw: If you want to be heard, you have to open your mouth and drop your jaw for the voice to come out. Lightly place your fingertips on your jaw joint (in front of your ear) and yawn. Sense the space under your fingertips enlarging as the jaw drops down. Practice speaking feeling the jaw move down and up as you speak. Look in a mirror and observe whether your jaw is opening and closing or if it is in a fixed high position.

b. Tongue: If your tongue is lazy, your articulation will be careless. Trace your tongue's movement as you slowly speak this phrase: "tip of the tongue." On the "t's," feel your tongue touch the ridge behind your upper front teeth. Repeat this phrase with precision of placement and accelerated speed never allowing the "T's" to touch your teeth.

c. Palate: This soft muscle at the back of your throat with a hanging appendage (uvula) is responsible for sending your voice out your nose or out your mouth. If your voice is nasal, get your soft palate muscle toned up. Looking into a mirror, observe your palate moving up as you yawn or sing "ah." Practice lifting your palate on a sustained "ah" and holding the lifted position for the count of ten. Repeat this exercise to develop muscle strength.

d. Lips: Your voice tends to die on your lips if you fail to activate and shape your lips as you speak. Watch TV reporters and anchors and observe lips that are engaged and those that are not. Get your lips moving by shaping them for the phrase, "Hello, how are you?" Next, whisper the same phrase keeping the lip shaping. Finally, speak the phrase with exaggerated lip activity. Use a mirror and observe your lip action.

5. Use an appealing voice quality: Using an attractive voice quality grabs and keeps the attention of your listener. The appealing voice makes optimum use of the vocal process: the breath is free, the throat is open, the resonators are mixed and the articulation is clear without distracting speech habits and thick accents. It also seduces the listener with its quality and uses a variety of volume, rate and pitch changes.

Avoid using the following vocal qualities. They are unattractive to many ears and some demonstrate vocal misuse or abuse.

a. Nasal: This is a whining sound that makes you sound like a complainer. People are likely to think nothing ever pleases you! The voice leaks up into your nose when it should be using your mouth as the exit. The lazy muscle at the back of your throat (the soft palate) is the cause of nasality. The palate fails to close off the passage leading to your nose. All speech sounds should flow out of your mouth except for the three nasal consonants: m, n, ng.

TIP: *Lightly place your fingertips on the bridge of your nose and monitor for the absence of vibrations as you slowly speak this sentence: "Every little boy ate a bite of bread."*

b. Denasal: If you sound as if you always have a stuffy nose or a cold in your head, your voice is denasal. This voice doesn't carry well because it's difficult to get the nasal sounds (m, n, ng) into the nose. Allergies, a deviated septum, or an obstruction contribute to this quality.

TIP: *Again, place your fingers lightly on the bridge of your nose. This time, encourage an abundance of vibrations on every m, n, ng. Speak the following sentence lengthening the nasal consonants: "Many women make much money."*

c. *Harsh:* Women who try to lower their voices often end up sounding harsh. Because they are compressing their vocal folds and pushing down on their voice, they tend to be judged as being overly aggressive. Moving your voice down in pitch also can be injurious to your vocal folds.

TIP: *Keep your voice out of "the basement" and your breath flowing as you speak.*

d. *Strident:* Women are frequently accused of being strident when more frequently, their voices are strident. The strident voice sounds high and shrill. The voice box (larynx) rides up the throat like an elevator when the speaker gets emotional.

TIP: *Place your fingertips on your adam's apple, yawn and feel its decent. Yawn the apple down whenever your voice moves high in pitch.*

e. *Throaty:* This back of the throat, "plumy" quality sounds as if you are talking down a cardboard tube. Others might think you are trying to put on airs. The tongue pulls back into the throat, thereby creating abundant throat resonance. Coaching addresses forward tone focus and appropriate tongue shaping of vowels.

TIP: *Make a motorboat sound with your breath, voice and lips. Once you've got your engine going (your breath and voice flowing), motorboat into speaking this line: "Hello, how are you?" Let your motorboat ride into "hello." Keep your voice moving through this entire exercise.*

f. *Thin:* Thinness is heard in the adolescent, so avoid this quality if you are over fifteen! It's weak in volume, sounds submissive, and suggests a lack of confidence. The jaw is held high and the voice resonates primarily in the mouth. This voice needs chest resonance!

TIP: *Place the palm of your hand on your chest bone and sustain "ah" in a yawn position. Monitor and encourage vibrations on your hand—feel the purr! Maintain these vibes as you speak.*

g. *Chesty:* Women who have to compete with men may believe they have to sound like them and thus adopt this vocal quality. This voice is abnormally low in pitch, resonates in the chest, lacks ring and is sometimes mistaken for a male voice. The chesty, or pectoral, voice needs more top.

TIP: *Speak for three minutes in your falsetto voice—the one you had when you were a kid. Your voice will sounds very high and make you feel a bit silly. Remain in your falsetto vice using lots of breath. Your tone will be somewhat airy. After three minutes, walk your voice down in pitch to where you like it. With practice you will sense that perhaps your pitch has not changed, but that your voice now has more brightness, overtones and ring.*

h. *Aspirate:* Marilyn Monroe and Jacqueline Kennedy Onassis used this breathy, semi-whispered quality. Some voice users like this quality because they feel it is sensually seductive; others may use it because they may not want to really be heard. The vocal folds do not come together completely and air escapes between the folds. It's difficult to project with a breathy voice.

TIP: *Belly breathing, supporting your voice as in singing, and simply wanting to be heard can discourage aspiration.*

    i. Husky or hoarse: This voice is in distress and may be suffering from misuse, abuse, or gastric reflux. If you tighten or strain your voice, talk a lot, scream and shout, your voice may become husky or hoarse. The edges of your vocal folds no longer come together with smooth edges, thus producing an unclear tone.

TIP: *Avoid screaming, shouting, straining and smoking. Speak softly and rest your voice until clear tone returns. If it doesn't return, seek out an ear, nose and throat specialist for an evaluation. Also, read the tips on "How to Keep your Voice Healthy."*

6. Modulate volume levels: The expressive voice uses all volume levels. The insecure voice tens to use low volume while a bravado voice may select only high volume. Others are guilty of using fading volume. The speaker using this behavior begins speaking with full voice but fades out at the end of a sentence. Fading volume suggests that the last words in the sentence are not important.

TIP: *Avoid speaking louder than the noise in a room, but enjoy using a full volume range when expressing high emotional moments. However, you can best express yourself if you have a handle on volume gradation.*

7. *Vary your speaking rate:* Let your breath (not your head) determine your speaking rate. Take frequent pauses and vary their lengths. Speak in phrases, ideas or logical segments. Be aware of your listener's response to your message. The response lets you know if you should talk faster, talk slower, or stop talking.

TIP: *If you tend to be a run-on speaker, wait for your breath to drop in before speaking. Lie on the floor on your belly and prop yourself up on your elbows. In this position you can feel your breath move your belly into the floor. Read aloud from a newspaper waiting each time for your breath. Breathe when you need to instead of at the end of your sentence.*

8. *Play the melody in your voice:* Enjoy full pitch range—all the notes you have in your voice. If you can sing them, you can speak them! Extending your pitch range shows that you are flexible and not afraid of risking. Your voice will also sound energetic.

TIP: *Sing a phrase or line of your favorite song. Breathe and speak the same phrase or line, allowing your voice to travel the same melodic distance. Continue using this sing/speak technique through the entire song. Tape and replay your final tape and assess.*

With the new options you've just explored, you are beginning to bring out the best of your voice and its special sound. Discovering your own voice is an exciting journey. It means giving up old habits that no longer reflect who we are and risking and exploring new options that better fit our goals today.

There is also sheer sensory pleasure in the sound and vibrations of your voice as they transverse your body and thrill your ear. The sound of your voice can make you and those with whom you speak feel what you are feeling: happy or sad, energetic or exhausted, etc. The big deal here is that you are in charge of the choices you make. You are the final arbitrator of how you want to sound and how you want to be perceived.

Lucille Schutmaat Rubin, Ph.D., director of Professionally Speaking in New York City, is a voice, speech and media coach who has helped many women find their voices. Her clients include executives, performers, speakers and TV personalities. She presents seminars and workshops throughout the United States and abroad and has authored many articles on vocal image and public speaking.

Hair

By Anthony Sorensen

Your hairstyle is an ongoing expression throughout life of one's own personal style. It expresses how one feels about oneself and how we want to be perceived by the world. Maintaining hair's health and vitality is important at any age. Through years of experience in the hair industry, I have seen many common mistakes made by women that can be easily avoided. Remember, natural looking is always more beautiful.

Of utmost importance, is to choose a hairstylist and colorist. Find a professional whose own personal style is similar to yours. Book a consultation or even book a few, they are free. Ask your stylist questions like where they were trained, how many years experience they have, and with whom they have worked. Choose a stylist who takes the time to ask you questions as well. Your lifestyle, what you do for a living, and your at-home styling regime will determine the best haircut for you. If you see a style that you like on a woman, ask where she had it done. Any woman is flattered by such a gesture. If a particular hairstyle in a magazine catches your eye, cut it out and bring it. As I always tell my clients, a picture is worth a thousand words. If you feel comfortable, book a haircut. Comfortable means asking questions at any time during a haircut—it's your money. Also, any good stylist can make your hair look like a magazine cover that day. Make sure it's a style you can do yourself at home. If there's a particular technique your stylist uses, be sure to ask him/her to not only show you, but do it yourself in their presence. I always put blow dryer, brush, roller or whatever tool I'm using, in my own clients' hand to help improve their technique. This way you'll feel more comfortable doing it yourself when time is of the essence.

How you style your hair on your own can make or break the cut you've just gotten. Be patient with yourself and remember practice makes perfect. With so many styling products available, one can get overwhelmed. Find out what your stylist used and go from there. Some safeguard formulas and sure-fire tricks of my own are as follows: For natural curly hair you want to control the frizz while accentuating the curl, mix a non-alcohol gel with a hydrating cream. Don't be stingy with the amount of product. Apply to soaking wet hair, comb through, then shake hair up from the roots without running fingers through. Don't touch until dry whether diffused or on its own - too much touching while wet causes frizz. Then shake up again. Natural means just that—*natural*. So let it be.

When blowing hair straight, use a straightening balm, a large boar bristle round brush, and a dryer equipped with a nozzle. Always take manageable sections depending on the size of your brush. Get the root dry first and follow through to the ends. Don't forget, hair becomes straight at the root, so don't be afraid of a little tension. And remember ladies, placing wet hair on hair that's already dry makes for come-back curls or waves.

Knowing every girl needs a little volume, Velcro rollers and a touch of volumizing spray goes a long way. Set dry section with a little volumizer at the root. When setting the roller, over direct the root, meaning set your roller a little bit forward from the section of hair. Now go do your makeup and get dressed. Then ensure your hair is set by going over it with a cool shot before taking out the rollers. After all, the cool button on the dryer is meant for more than just cooling yourself off in the bathroom. Presto!—instant volume. And never ever go back into the hair with heat once the volume is created because hair is set in the cooling process.

For over processed damaged hair, my biggest recommendation is to not wash your hair as much. I guarantee just cutting your washing to every second or third day will dramatically change the texture of your hair. Our hair needs the natural oils we produce. Wet and style as much as you like, just don't wash it all the time. Washing your hair too often causes your scalp to overproduce oil, so a three to four week adjustment period will be necessary, but I promise, worthwhile.

A common question I'm always asked is "when am I too old for long hair?" With aging, unfortunately, our whole body slows down, including the hair follicle. The diameter of the hair becomes finer and length becomes shorter. So at a certain age, a shorter haircut can make hair less prone to looking limp and lifeless. It's an individual decision based on the condition of one's own hair as determined by genetics. I have clients in their fifties with more beautiful long hair than some of my clients in their twenties. So if your hair is healthy and your attitude is young, I say go for it.

Most stylists would and should trim your bangs for free. But if your busy schedule can't afford a visit to the salon, you and I both know, you're going to break out those cuticle scissors to do a number on them yourself. So try this: When bangs are wet, take a small section of your bangs and twist them. Slice downward with your scissors starting at a length longer than the intended length you desire, because dry hair will spring up. Then when dry, trim across cutting only the longest hairs. Remember, longer is always safer.

We all know bad hair days, so when the air is extra thick, your umbrella got caught in the wind, or the convertible top won't come up, make sure you've kept a few Velcro rollers, some volumizer, or hydrating cream in your bag. Also, that nozzle on the hand dryer in the restroom is adjustable you know. So stop in for a midday pick-me-up, your hair will thank you for it.

In this day and age, a woman doesn't have to be afraid of showing sensuality with her hair. Day or night, in the office or on the street, choose a style that brings out the best in you. Taking the time to style your hair proves more beneficial to mood and self-esteem than a trip to the shrink. So have fun with your hair, try new styles—experiment. Arrive in style and with confidence, always presenting your best hair forward. It will show in your attitude and presence.

Anthony Sorensen was trained at the Frederic Fekkai salon in Manhattan. He has been featured in W *magazine, dailycandy.com, and* The London Times. *He has been part of the team for makeovers on "Live with Regis and Kathie Lee," and "The Maury Povich Show." He is frequently called upon by his discreet clientele list to travel as far as London Monaco, St Simon's Island, and Los Angeles. His editorial work can be seen in both national and international publications.*

ACKNOWLEDGEMENTS

First, thanks to my incredible husband, Henry Rosenberg, who has so enriched my life, whom I love so dearly, and who has renewed my faith in men.

Thanks to my wonderful children, Adam and Alexandra who make my life so rich and wonderful. Though not without a few heart-wrenching moments!

To my wonderful nephew Jason and his wife Chi and the memory of his mother and my sister, who died four years ago.

To Mariette Hartley, who I love like my sister, who gave me her love, her friendship and belief in my talent to land my job working with her on the CBS Morning Show. Those were such wonderful days.

To my dearest, most wonderful friends, Debra Refson and Judith Gray, who help me realize every day how important the power of friendship is for women.

To my wonderful friend Mary Ellen for always being there for me and helping to save my life in so many ways.

To Patty Sicular, my booker at the Ford Modeling Agency who always believed in me and got me through those amazing days as a model. I love you Patty, and you will always be in my life.

To all the wonderful people at Paraview Press who believed in me and my book and have been there for me all the way. Erika Lieberman and Claire Wyckoff, I couldn't have done it without you!

And finally, to Andrea Thompson who made this book happen. You are truly wonderful. Thank you and your great husband, Bill, for all your help.

www.ingramcontent.com/pod-product-compliance
Lightning Source LLC
Chambersburg PA
CBHW020244290326
41930CB00038B/250